AND THE SUN IS UP:
KUNDALINI RISES IN THE WEST

AND THE SUN IS UP:
KUNDALINI RISES IN THE WEST

by

W. Thomas Wolfe

For seekers of self.
For those who are more than
curious about psychic phenomena
and spiritual or mystical experiences.

SUN BOOKS
Sun Publishing Company

Copyright ©1978 by W. Thomas Wolfe
Reprinted through arrangements with Academy Hill
Press, origninal publishers.
First printing, May 1978
First Sun Books Printing,   May 1987

SUN BOOKS
are published by
SUN PUBLISHING COMPANY
P.O. Box 5588
Santa Fe, NM
87502-5588

ISBN: 0-89540-166-5

Printed in the United States of America

Dedication

To Al and R.M. But mostly, to Sue, Tommy, and Robbie, without whose understanding this volume would not exist.

Acknowledgements

My deepest appreciation to all those kind friends and loved ones who helped me with this volume. Specifically, thanks to R.M. for his literary edit of my first draft; thanks also to James (Barney) Bornn for his excellent photos; thanks to Alice Mansfield, without whose efficient typing this book would still be in draft form; and thanks to my wife, Sue, for her careful readings of and comments on my early material.

INTRODUCTION TO THE SUN BOOKS EDITION

It's been ten years since the Kundalini event described in this book took place. Measured in some ways, ten years is a very long time. But in terms of the Kundalini event, it has been but a moment for me, with the wonder of the orginal event and period immediately before and after the event still resounding within me. Nevertheless, time cures us all, just as surely as smoking cures the hanging ham; and both my lifestyle and thought on Kundalini have matured over the intervening years.

Between 1975 and 1980 I reflected a great deal on what Kundalini is: why the classic "symptoms" affect some people but not others, the various degrees of Kundalini activity, the relation of the Kundalini effects to experiences encountered in some of the more exoteric religous practices. Some answers I found, while others eluded me. Ultimately, though, I realized that reflection on Kundalini — even by one who has experienced the classical Kundalini event — is a product of the small "i" looking for some edge over the rules and laws of earthly existence. And the only hope for true spiritual integration is to give up, naturally and in one's own time, the chase for spiritual superiority, measured righteousness, and other characteristics that set man off from man in our materialistic world.

Dr. Lee Sannella, author of *Kundalini: Psychosis or Transcendence,* once spoke of the "essential benign, beneficient, and deeply intelligent character" of Kundalini. Indeed, Kundalini knows everything it needs to know about itself, just as one's body knows everything fundamental to its operation —how to breathe, how to grow, how to suckle, how to die. So, too, does the truly spiritual person know everything about being spiritual that he or she needs to know. For one who truly lives in grace, reflections on spirituality, morality, and other such topics, including Kundalini, are necessary only to point out to others who want to "know." Reflections and judgements, while necessary when dealing with issues of morality and unessential knowledge, are simply not a fundamental part of being spiritual.

The Kundalini experience, while perhaps an indicator of one who is on the way to self-knowledge, does not in itself make one a spiritually integrated person. Nor are the classical Kundalini experience and enlightenment necessarily concurrent. Furthermore, one does not necessarily need the classical Kundalini experience in order to become enlightened. To find the way, one need only give up the search, as we have so often been told.

Nevertheless, the Kundalini experience *is* one of the most important, impressive, personality-changing and lifestyle-changing events that one can experience. And, because it can be one of the most traumatic (and even painful) events in your life, it is comforting to know how and why it happens, and what to expect when it does —information which you will find in this book.

Now, what about the years since 1980? Simply put, my intellectual reflections on Kundalini have taken a back seat to living life. I've learned that it's OK to express preferences, OK to enjoy the products of our world, OK to get on with enjoying the life that hums within. But it's OK to reflect, too. So, if you are interested in Kundalini, if you have a burning desire to know who and what you are and what you are doing in this world, if you want to know more about psychic phenomena, then read on.

Your search has taken you to a most interesting book, one which will hopefully help you find the way on the path to knowing yourself.

W. Thomas Wolfe
November 1985

Contents

Prologue 9
Introduction 11

PART 1: Kundalini Them

The Hindu's View 15
  The Kundalini Promise 15
  The Kundalini Mechanism 16
  Ingredients of the Concoction 19
The Exoteric Christian's View 23
  The Christian Promise 23
  The Christian Mechanism 23
  Ingredients of the Concoction 24
The Esoteric Christian's View 27
  The Mystic Christian Promise 27
  The Mystic Christian Mechanism 27
The Professional Specialist's View 29
The Kundalini Subject's View 33
  Physiological Effects 34
  Spiritual Weightlessness 41
  Celibacy and Other Austerities 42
  Emotional and Attitudinal Changes 42
  Changed Dream Content 44
  Awareness of the Internal/External
    Servomechanism 46
  The "Satsang" Effect 47
  Concept and Paradox Resolution 48
  Event Control 50
  Control of the Force 50
  The Total Effect 52
A Summary of Part One 54

PART 2: Kundalini Me

Prologue to Part Two 57
The Setup 63
Preliminary Experiences 67
  Experimenting with Meditation 68

The Biofeedback Machine 69
Attainment Dreams 71
Some Stronger Early Warnings 76
The "Feelie": A Psychic Gift From Kundalini 78
The Kundalini Awakening 81
Ka-boom! 83
The Validation 86
Aftermath: The Next Seven Months 93
Injury (Modification) to Right-Brain 93
Possession Attempts 95
Descent of the White Light 99
Trying Out the New Controls 100
A New Player: A Collective Consciousness 104
The Conflagration 108
New Kundalini Symptoms 113
The Sun Is Up: Visions of the Blue Bindu 120
Reintegration 123
And Today 124
Some Afterthoughts 129

PART 3: Kundalini You

Prologue to Part Three 137
Invoking the Kundalini 139
The Reason for Summoning the Kundalini 139
Obstacles to the Kundalini Awakening 142
Removing the Obstacles 146
Formal Practice 159

PART 4: Kundalini We

Speculation on the Growth of a Collective
Kundalini 163
Christ and the Kundalini 164
Kundalini and the Second Coming 167
A Modern Parallel to the Second Coming 169

Appendix A: Biofeedback and Kundalini
Arousal 177
Bibliography 182

PROLOGUE

This book tells about an individual and collective psychic event, called a "Kundalini awakening," that is currently taking place with increasing frequency across the world.

The experience, a quickening of vital forces now lying nearly dormant in man, flamed on with startling intensity for the author early in 1975. It was to change his view completely of who and what he and other men are, and of what is possible in the normally perceived universe of linear time and space.

The Kundalini experience is not new. Under one name or another, it has been sought by spiritual adventurers for thousands of years. And although the name "Kundalini" has not yet been heard by many Western ears, esoteric Kundalini concepts underlie many of the Biblical teachings of Christianity, as well as teachings of other major religions.

There are many ways to describe it: the Kundalini awakening; enlightenment; salvation; Christ Consciousness; the coming of the dove—and it will be said in all of these ways in this book. But the experience itself has common physiological roots, no matter what approach to religion is taken or what specific cultural manifestations result from the quickening of the vital forces.

When Kundalini rises in man, it magnifies all of his internal traits: it brings to the surface the best and worst of him. Because of this, it behooves the Kundalini aspirant to make a better person of himself. Those who approach the Kundalini with the right attitude can be transformed into mental and spiritual giants simply by surrendering to the natural forces within. But those who are not ready, those who are poor of kindness and compassion but who nevertheless go on to force the Kundalini into wakefulness, can be crushed, mentally and physically, by the iron hand of their own shortcomings.

Kundalini is not only an individual phenomenon, but also a collective one: it moves today in the world around us. The time is coming when it will be impossible for man to resist the collective pullings of the Kundalini. In these times, the war between higher spirit and materialism will be waged in and around each of us. Great beings of the past who were familiar with Kundalini phenomena were able to comfortably predict that this would happen because they could see the workings of the experience within themselves. The Kundalini phenomenon, the second coming, the aquarian age — all of these are the same. And they are upon us.

Here then is a fresh view of ancient knowledge, told through personal experience of Kundalini. This book is meant to turn on lights in the unfamiliar hallways that many of you will soon walk.

INTRODUCTION

Kundalini has been revered in esoteric circles, primarily in the Eastern world, for thousands of years. Until just a few years ago, Kundalini incidents were scattered lightly across the ages. Great spiritual leaders like Guatama the Buddha, Christ, Mohammed, Moses,—these and others like them* were privileged to be "in this world but not of it."

All of these great beings were initiated by the firey Kundalini. And they experienced subsequent realities that were not available to the men left untouched by Kundalini.

But now, especially in the spiritually-hungry West, the Kundalini phenomenon is spreading rapidly, absorbing all those it finds ready into its fold. It seems that man's need to know God and self in his super-hectic society has acted as a signal fire in attracting the process to him.

The process is highly contagious. Kundalini now affects barbers, plumbers, assembly line personnel, disk jockeys, waitresses, computer programmers, and others from all walks of life.

Even while you read this book, Kundalini will rise within you if you release yourself to it. And once the process is started, there is no return. Once the current has flown through your body, the internal changes are set in motion.

Neurologically, the man or woman struck by Kundalini will be transformed into a different creature. The autonomic and central nervous systems will eventually be united under conscious control. Right hemisphere and left hemisphere physiology will be more closely coordinated than in the normal person. These changes will permit the new man to see unity within himself and within the universe around him.

But those who undergo the experience will need to make the greatest sacrifice of all, and of this you must be fore-

*Re: "Cosmic Consciousness," by R. Bucke

warned: you will sacrifice your small self to share in the joys of the larger entity, the higher being within you. You will be a drop of water becoming the ocean.

To be an advanced being means giving up all those things you think you are. At every level of your being your psychic footholds, your personal characteristics, your concepts, and your beliefs about self and reality, will disintegrate. You will need to let God, the higher being within you, run rampant through you.

And now, a little about what to expect in this book: Part 1, Kundalini Them, reviews what the Kundalini is in the Hindu tradition. It also describes what the Kundalini means to modern professional and religious groups, and what it means to the typical modern-day person struck by the Kundalini awakening. This orientation should help you to understand what the Kundalini is and how to react to similar inner stirrings within you.

Part 2, Kundalini Me, describes my Kundalini awakening and how I was affected. It includes some information on my background, tells how Kundalini struck, explains what happened afterward, and describes how my dreams helped me assimilate the total experience. Where applicable, I provide analysis of my experience to compare what happened to me to the traditional view of travel on the spiritual path.

Part 3, Kundalini You, describes what you should do to prepare yourself for the experience. This information will help you make your transition safely.

Part 4, Kundalini We, is a model for the future. It ties together the Kundalini phenomenon, the concept of the second coming, and evolution of man into a higher being.

Before proceeding into Part 1, I want to admit to the same shortcoming that occurs in all who experience the Kundalini awakening. That is, each subject translates the event into terms and concepts with which he is familiar and comfortable. All spiritual concepts, for example, are meaningful on an individual basis only, and as a result will appear subjective to those who do not naturally follow the same beliefs. If there are passages with which you do not agree, do not reject them out of hand. Instead, I urge you to look for the deeper meaning as it applies to your religion, your beliefs, and your personal values in life.

PART 1: KUNDALINI THEM

THE HINDU'S VIEW

Esoteric Hindu scriptures describe a serpent-like force that resides coiled at the base of the spine. This force, known as *Kundalini, Kundalini Shakti, Chiti Shakti,* and various other Hindu terms, is referred to as "Kundalini" throughout this book.

The Kundalini lies dormant, sleeping with one eye open, so to speak, stirring only infrequently, and then gently, during the lives of most people. It is said that Kundalini is the force drawn from mother earth that makes one alive, and that even the infrequent and greatly reduced activity evidenced in the vast majority of people is enough to carry each being through an intelligent, vital life on earth.

The ancients discovered that the sleeping Kundalini could be aroused by certain techniques. They also discovered that to do this was indeed a highly dangerous undertaking. They found that the body must be ready to accept the Kundalini awakening, and that if the awakening was rushed, severe damage would sometimes result to the seeker's body and psyche.

They found, for example, that in some unfortunate cases men would go mad. And all kinds of distressing ailments would happen to their physical bodies. In some very violent cases, it is said, men would be spirited completely out of this world with an accompanying clap of thunder and a wisp of quickly disappearing smoke.

But as strange as it may seem, neither this violent exit from the known world nor the prospect of madness was a deterrent to the ever-present line of Kundalini seekers. What was it that drove men to welcome potential annihilation with open arms?

The Kundalini Promise

The answer, of course, is that the potential fruits of success outweigh the pains of failure. When successful, the end result of the Kundalini awakening, usually some years later, is enlightenment—self-realization.

When one is enlightened, one gets to know who he really is. He becomes one with all that is, and there are no more problems for him—no more suffering, no more searching for identity.

In Hindu belief, the enlightened man is eventually absorbed into the formless aspect of God—Nirvana. He is removed from the cyclic wheel of birth, death, and rebirth. He has "gotten it right" and has gone home to God. In some cases, the liberated one remains in human form to minister to the less fortunate and lead them to what is now his. The Hindus believe this to be a great sacrifice on his part—to remain embodied on earth when he could otherwise be absorbed into God. Such a being is highly respected and is called a *Jivanmukti.*

In addition to enlightenment, there are secondary benefits. (And in many cases, the secondary benefits are the ones that start the searcher on the path.) A Kundalini-awakened individual will usually develop *Siddhi* (powers) not normally available to the ordinary man. For example, some develop advanced intellects; some can see forward in time; some can move objects without touching them; some develop healing powers; some read minds; and some receive all of these gifts and more.

But the primary goal is self-realization. The other benefits are to be enjoyed and used wisely, but not exalted. To misuse or exalt these powers, say the texts, will delay the progress toward self-realization and plunge the seeker back into darkness.

The Kundalini Mechanism

According to Hindu tradition, the Kundalini lies coiled in 3 1/2 loops in an area called the *Kanda* at the base of the spine. When the Kundalini begins to awaken, it travels up the spine, uncoiling as it goes. The route taken is through a central *nadi* (nerve channel) called the *Sushumna.* The *Sushumna* is a hollow channel encompassing and running the length of the spine into the head.

There are two other nerve channels, the *Ida* and *Pingala,* which also run the length of the spine, criss-crossing back and forth and forming a pattern with the *Sushumna* similar to the physician's caduceus.

An ideal awakening is one in which the *Sushumna, Ida,* and *Pingala* transport a balanced flow of the Kundalini force to the head. In some unfortunate cases, the Kundalini is diverted into either the *Ida* or *Pingala* channel, rather than running through all three channels in a balanced fashion. In these instances, searing pain and other unpleasant manifestations result.*

As the Kundalini proceeds upward, it passes through esoteric nerve plexuses called *chakras*. As it reaches each of these seven *chakras* in the body, the Kundalini pierces it, causing manifestations associated with the specific *chakra*.

The first *chakra*, located just above the anus, is associated with survival drives. The second *chakra*, slightly higher, is associated with sex. The third *chakra*, located at the base of the rib cage, is associated with vitality and drive to power. The fourth *chakra*, the heart *chakra*, is the first of the spiritually "higher" *chakras*. It is associated with compassion and love. The fifth, or throat *chakra*, is the energy center. Through this *chakra* energy passes to and from the body. The sixth *chakra* is sometimes referred to as the "third eye." It is linked with psychic phenomena and heightened mental powers. The seventh *chakra* is found at the top of the head. Called the "Crown *Chakra*", or *Sahasrar*, this *chakra* is associated with spiritual man. It is the link between man's higher self and his lower self. When the Kundalini reaches the

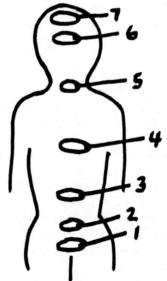

* Re: *"Kundalini: The Evolutionary Energy in Man,"* by Gopi Krishna, published by Shambhala.

seventh *chakra* it unites with the *Atman* (higher self) within man. After this mystic marriage has occurred, the individual is enlightened.

The time it takes Kundalini to make the trip from the first to the seventh *chakra* can vary greatly, depending on the attitude and physiological condition of the initiate at the time the Kundalini first stirs. In the "classical" awakening, the entire trip is made very rapidly, within minutes, or even seconds. In these cases, all the *chakras* are pierced in rapid order, and the event is accompanied by a plethora of unusual and sometimes frightening phenomena. The classical awakening does not usually energize the *chakras* permanently. After the classical awakening the *chakras* will usually be taken again, one by one, over a three to twelve year cycle. The final result, it is said, is permanent bliss, super-intelligence for some, psychic powers for some, but most of all, oneness with all that is.

There are many variations to the mechanics behind Kundalini. Some factions say there are six *chakras;* others say there are as many as 13 of these "many-petaled lotuses." Some followers say that there is a downward flow, or return trip of Kundalini, before the event is consumated. Other countries and religions approach the event under their own traditions and cultural belief structures. In any event, the *Sushumna, Ida, Pingala, Kanda,* and *Chakra* systems are esoteric devices that do not exist in the physical body, but are provided through antiquity to explain the unusual internal feelings experienced by people in whom the Kundalini has begun to rise. There are many excellent books to which the reader can refer for a more detailed study of the esoteric mechanics of Kundalini.

When the Kundalini is awakened, spontaneous side-effects are noticed. For example, vigorous involuntary breathing patterns can develop; the body of the initiate can jerk about violently as he sits in a meditative state; his body might assume various postures without being directed to do so; he might lose his desire for sex during certain phases of the experience; he might develop a devotional attitude toward his choice of diety; he might seem to understand paradoxical concepts that others cannot understand; and he might occasionally withdraw into meditative *Samadhi,* a state of nearly unconscious bliss.

These side-effects are, of course, noticed by others desiring to rouse the Kundalini. It is not difficult to see, here,
that the cart could very easily be put before the horse by
excited seekers. And in fact this is the case. All of the various
yogas, or spiritual disciplines, use techniques that emphasize
the side-effects as a means to get to the experience. But
while Kundalini causes these spontaneous effects, it is not
evident that practicing the effects will gain the experience.

In trying to invoke Kundalini, many Eastern advocates go
to extreme lengths. Some, for example, vow celibacy for the
remainder of their lives. Others give away all their worldly
possessions, not understanding that renunciation is an attitudinal change and not a material change. Others sit in silence
for the rest of their lives; others find caves and die there;
still others put their bodies through incredible tortures to
prove that they are beyond the body. None of these extremes
is necessary.

Ingredients of the Concoction

There are a number of concepts woven into the Kundalini
brew that have correlations in other religions and practices
that do not necessarily recognize the Kundalini phenomenon
by its Hindi name. Since I will be discussing some of the
similarities of Kundalini and Christian concepts in the next
chapter, I will briefly cover some of the Hindu ingredients
here.

The Guru: The term "guru" means one who brings light
where there was darkness before. In Hindu tradition, there
are lineages of great beings who have incarnated on earth
to help mankind know himself. These are the gurus.

The Hindus feel that approaching the Kundalini on one's
own is too dangerous, that one could too easily get lost on
the path. To prevent this from happening, the guru, one
who has been there, becomes the focus for the devotion of
his followers. He acts as a surrogate God to help his devotees
know God themselves.

Surrender: The guru's main ploy is to get the devotee to the
point where he has complete faith in the guru. When this
happens, the devotee surrenders his life, his being, to the

guru. When this total surrender takes place, the guru ex-
cites the devotee's Kundalini into rising through his body,
thereby causing the enlightenment cycle to begin. This is
initiation by fire.

The whole idea of the guru/devotee relationship is that
surrender to the external guru will act subliminally to permit
true surrender to the devotee's own higher being within him.

Adverse Forces: Kundalini followers believe that adverse,
or "dark," forces will swoop upon the man on the path,
attempting to test his mettle and sway him from the path
if he is not yet physically or mentally ready for enlightenment. Kundalini followers believe that all is God. Therefore,
the adverse forces must also be part of God, provided to
moderate the Kundalini subject's speed along the path. Many
believe that without the suffering caused by the adverse
forces people would become comfortable in their unaware-
ness of self, never desiring to advance closer to God.

It seems that the adverse forces can work two ways: some
people can be goaded, through suffering, into seeking something better, while others can be frightened, through their
own as yet unpurged fear and greed, into abandoning the
path until they have learned more about compassion and
have worked on making themselves better people. Actually,
both types are being helped toward God at the level of
their own needs and desires, and at a speed they can handle.

Ignorance: Until a man is awakened, say the Hindus, he
lives in a fantasy world of *maya* (illusion). He assumes that
the attributes and values he assigns to things are as real as
the things themselves, when intrinsically these attributes and
values have no reality other than being a projection of the
one who perceives.

A man living in *maya* evaluates things in matched pairs
such as bad versus good; beautiful versus ugly; intelligent
versus stupid; like versus dislike, high versus low. This evalu-
ation, which must always be relative, colors the true reality of
the perceived object to the extent that the object can no
longer be seen as it is. And the sleeper applies this dualistic
thinking to everything: it is you (or it) and me; we and they;
them and us.

When man awakens, according to the Hindus, he simply

remembers who he really is. He no longer sets himself apart from the rest of the universe. A digression is in order here: Imagine, if you will, a hypothetical beginning of time in which an enormous cloud of pure being exists, filling all space. Soon some movement begins to stir within. As the movement intensifies, dense pockets of matter begin to condense within the cloud. It is here where illusion begins: as objects are formed, relationships arise because the dense forms begin to sense a difference between "themselves" and the rest of all that is. They begin to perceive in special ways, and thereby begin to accept or reject what they see. They love and relate, or they reject and dissociate. Although the life within them still belongs to the larger being, they begin the long journey away from knowledge of self and toward individuation.

The more a man thinks he is an individual apart from God, the more he falls from grace and descends into ignorance, illusion. Ignorance, to the Hindu, is simply not remembering who you are. The situation is rectified by the Kundalini event.

THE EXOTERIC CHRISTIAN'S VIEW

The exoteric, or conventional, Christian* is in most cases not aware of the existence of Kundalini. Nevertheless, the Christian religion has the same spiritual superstructure that Kundalini tradition has. In fact, many of the events depicted in the Bible are almost literal descriptions of the Kundalini event. The Christ story, itself, parallels and symbolizes the Kundalini awakening by describing the transition of the "Son of Man" into the "Son of God." This is not unlike the Kundalini transition from normal, ego-ruled man into the self-realized being.

The Christian Promise

Christian tradition promises a heaven after death to those who are worthy and a hell to those who are not. Most Christians believe that to gain entrance to heaven, one must accept Jesus Christ as personal savior to intercede for man and lead him to God.

Christian tradition is not as rich as Hindu tradition in spelling out what the rewards of heaven will be. Instead, more emphasis is placed on having faith that heaven is desirable.

Christians believe that there will be a second coming of Christ — that Christ will gather all those who have accepted him, whether they be dead or alive, and take them home with him to God. This is not unlike the Hindu concept of rejoining the formless aspect of God and departing from the cycle of birth and death as man.

The Christian Mechanism

A few Christian denominations undergo Kundalini-like symptoms while in the grip of spiritual ecstasies. For example, some Christians "speak in tongues" during a high, spiritual-emotional state. Others will twist and turn, throw their hands

*My discussion of the conventional Christian is drawn from my own background of fundamental Protestant beliefs. Fundamental beliefs represent conservative Christianity and provide an excellent choice for comparison to the Kundalini concepts. Actually, there is a continuous spectrum of belief in the Christian tradition from fundamental through liberal and into mystic Christianity. The liberal/mystic range will be covered very briefly in the next chapter.

into the air, roll on the floor, and undergo other types of physical manifestations, but these are few. To most of Christianity, there are no physiological manifestations associated with basic beliefs.

The Christian mechanism is largely acceptance of Christ on **faith.** And the physiological effects noticed by the Kundalini followers are largely absent from exoteric Christianity.

While the idea of acceptance on faith is laudable, it is my opinion that it tends to externalize God—make him "other." As a result, the Christian tends to deal with God vicariously, as almost everything else is dealt with in Western society. Because of this, the total giving over to God within, which in Kundalini tradition is accompanied by strong, physiological manifestations, is not usually seen within the framework of Christianity. Therefore, the development of an esoteric mechanism to explain the effect has not been necessary.

Ingredients of the Concoction

Nevertheless, at a deeper level the Kundalini story is evident in the Bible. Many of the Christian concepts parallel the esoteric Hindu concepts. Here are but a few.

Jesus: Some historians feel that Jesus' years prior to his illumination in the river Jordan took him to India and other places where Eastern traditions were prevalent. Perhaps these historians are correct: the similarities between the Kundalini phenomenon and the Biblical concepts taught by Christ are quite similar.

To the Hindu who is familiar with the Kundalini phenomenon, it is obvious that Christ experienced and assimilated a Kundalini awakening and then tried to pass his newfound knowledge on in terms that would be understood by his countrymen.

In other words, Christ was the Christian Guru.

Acceptance of Christ: Christ taught that the way to God was through him. Just as the Hindu guru acts as surrogate God, so does Christ. And acceptance of Christ is the same as **surrender** to the Hindu guru.

The Bible points out that Christ can baptize with the Holy

Spirit. This is very similar to the Hindu concept in which the guru initiates the devotee by awakening the Kundalini within him. In both cases the price is the same: the devotee must surrender to the guru, who himself has already seen God and now stands as the bridge for other men to cross over.

The Devil: The Christian concept of the devil is very like the Hindu concept of the adverse forces: both traditions recognize that all is not roses on the path to salvation.

Unfortunately, the Christian concept of the devil has built-in limitations that most likely prevent the average Christian from experiencing the physiological rewards that are otherwise available to him. For example, the Bible refers to the devil as "the Angel of Light." This means that any experience of internal light or other unfamiliar symptoms are likely to be quickly shut off by the conventional Christian, rather than encouraged.

Further, unlike the Hindu concept in which the adverse forces act to moderate man's travel on the path, the Christian's concept sees the devil as antagonistic to, and different from, God. To the Christian, it is not the devil's work to moderate his advance along the path, but to win his soul to eternal damnation.

Sin: Just as the Hindu's basic condition is **ignorance,** the Christian's basic condition is sin. The Kundalini follower is awakened from ignorance; the Christian is purged of sin — both of these through acceptance of the guru.

In man's beginning, according to the Bible, Adam ate of the tree of knowledge of good and evil. He was then able to distinguish between bad and good. With this "knowledge", man opened the way to developing various guilts and other attitudinal deposits (known to the Hindus as "karma"). Although these new self-perceptions became very real burdens to the "sinful" man, they were nevertheless based in illusion.

The concept of discrimination as being man's original sin is quite similar to the concept of specialized perception that leads to individuation and separation from God, as discussed under "Ignorance" in the preceding chapter. Apparently, dualistic thinking, or the assignment of values to objects in the relative universe, is man's fall from Grace in both traditions.

THE ESOTERIC CHRISTIAN'S VIEW

The esoteric, or mystic, Christian is a person from a conventional Christian background who has studied and compared various religions and has assimilated personal interpretations and beliefs that are still Christian, but with Eastern overtones.

Many mystic Christians believe that until he turned 33 or thereabouts, Jesus was not yet the Christ: he was Jesus, son of the carpenter, Joseph. These Christians believe that while Jesus was being baptized in the river Jordan, he was approached by the dove and transformed into the Son of God.

Some mystics recognize Jesus' experience as a Kundalini event, while others maintain more standard, Christian interpretations. In any event, all believe that Jesus was possessed by a "Christ Consciousness" that is available to all who can find the key.

The Mystic Christian Promise

The mystic Christian believes that man can be enlightened, or transformed, while still alive, and thereby share in Christ's consciousness. The mystic Christian feels that the Christ Consciousness is already within everyone, and that it is but a matter of removing the blocks to this awareness to share in this consciousness. He believes that worship of Jesus Christ can bring the light of Christ Consciousness from the higher man within to the lower man.

The Mystic Christian Mechanism

The descriptions of internal activity offered by the mystic Christian begin to approach those of the Kundalini subject, indicating that physiological effects are in abundance within him. He will speak of such things as "white light" of a feeling of oneness welling up within him, but usually the affects he describes are not as mechanical as the Kundalini subject's description of the *chakra* system.

Christ Consciousness itself is usually preceded by a mystical experience or revelation of extreme intensity. This, of course, is very likely the same basic experience as the Kundalini event. The mystical experience is dictated by the individual's personal background and tendencies. For example, some will see a vision of Christ, the Mother Mary, or some other Christian saint. Others may have an impersonal, but overwhelming, feeling of unity, bliss, oneness with God.

Many mystics believe that the gates to heaven and hell are side by side, and that the mystical experience will maximize the most prominent tendencies in the one it strikes. Some say that if there is fear, greed, avarice, or other negative qualities in the heart, these will be magnified, and the smitten person will see his devils. But if the heart is filled with compassion, love, and acceptance, these are the qualities that are magnified.

There are many other analogies between the Kundalini experience and Christian teachings. Those that have been presented, however, should be enough to illustrate the point that the Kundalini experience, by whatever name, is deeply woven into the Bible, even though it is partially hidden in some of the exoteric interpretations. Expeditions into the sacred writings of other religions will find the Kundalini waiting there, as well.

THE PROFESSIONAL SPECIALIST'S VIEW

It is axiomatic that large changes are preceded by confusion, chaos, and other destructive events. The old order must first be disassembled to make space for the new.

So, too, with the Kundalini awakening. Kundalini treats roughest those aspirants having the greatest distance to travel — the greatest number of blocks to be removed. Where the advances of Kundalini are small and frequent, the seeker progresses relatively smoothly along the spiritual path with minimum disruption to his life style. But where the advances are large and infrequent, all of man's psychic buildings come tumbling down. No stone is left upon another. In such a case, every aspect of the initiate's psyche is shaken loose and blown away until it appears that surely there is nothing left to suffer.

The reason the effect is so sweeping is because the central nervous system and the brain — the human electrical system — are the parts of the body most intimately involved with the Kundalini awakening. And, of course, any large disturbance in the brain or the central nervous system will have unpredictable, far-reaching effects.

Because this effect is so inclusive, each of the various professional people brought in to cure the ailment will see symptoms relating to his particular specialty. For example, the neurologist will see nerve problems, some sort of nervous breakdown; the psychiatrist will see emotional and intellectual disorders — schizophrenia; the doctor will see various diseases and body disturbances that will usually turn out to be psychosomatic disorders or temporary physical disorders that go mysteriously into remission. Watching today's specialists try to cure a Kundalini "affliction" is like watching the blind men and the elephant, where each man tries to define the total elephant by the part he first happens upon.

In any case, the Western professional specialist, who by and large is not yet familiar with the Kundalini phenomenon, will see the awakening as a pathological occurrence — an illness; something to be treated with drugs, electro-shock therapy, institutionalization, or frontal lobotomy.

The person who is spontaneously struck by Kundalini, but is not aware of the phenomenon, is in trouble in such an environment. Not suspecting that the effects are due to a Kundalini awakening, he will generally pass from specialist to specialist, undergoing one atrocity after another in an attempt to purge himself of his curse. It is unlikely that he will come out unscathed.

The person who suspects that Kundalini is stirring should maintain his faith. Otherwise, he will walk a treacherous line between refusing treatment on one hand and seeking treatment on the other. He will worry that if he treats his condition with conventional methods, he will hinder or halt the progress of Kundalini, or divert it into some grotesque, unwanted variation. But on the other side of the coin, he is not certain that what he now feels is not pathological and perhaps requires medical or psychiatric treatment.

In the classical awakening, activity is first felt in the lower back.* This movement then slowly rises up the spine until it reaches the head. When the energy spills into the cranium, the subject experiences a magnification of emotions and other mental processes, as well as possible disruptions of body awareness and motor control. In some cases, the subject becomes oblivious of the external world, simply bathing in a pool of bliss and radiant light.

Some Western professionals are beginning to recognize the authenticity of the Kundalini phenomenon. Such a medical man would say that the central nervous system was somehow activated, first at the base of the spine and then spreading upward toward the base of the skull. This wave of energy traveling through the nerve bundles would act like a wave traveling through water, only in this case, it would travel up through the back. (It is not difficult to see how this effect can be likened to that of an uncoiling snake progressing up the spine.)

---

*Recent studies indicate that the movement sometimes begins in the feet and progresses up the legs before moving into the small of the back. The experience seems to vary from person to person.

Recently a new, exciting description of the "physio-Kundalini"* effect postulated a biological model that offers a logical explanation of why Kundalini behaves as it does. Very basically (and I request that you refer to the volumes mentioned in the footnote for a more complete explanation), electrical current travels from the brain stem upward through the center of the head, and then falls downward around the sides of the head, like a spout of water shooting straight up into the air and then spreading outward from the center as it falls back to earth. Electrical over-stimulation traveling this path would activate parts of the body in the order most usually experienced during the classical awakening.

Whether or not this effect is pathological is not a topic that will be discussed here at any length. The point is that the Kundalini phenomenon can now be explained from an up-to-date, neurological point of view, as well as from the more subjective, spiritual viewpoint.

---

*Refer to "Stalking the Wild Pendulum," by I. Bentov, Dutton publishers, and "Kundalini: Psychosis or Transcendence," by Lee Sannella, M.D., H. Dakin Publishers, for an interesting account of the physio-Kundalini effect.

THE KUNDALINI SUBJECT'S VIEW

Although the classical Kundalini awakening can take place without any advance warning, it usually happens after a few weeks of preliminary activity during which the subject has already noticed strange, new events in his life.

During this preliminary period, he may have begun to experience new aches and pains, or to hear strange sounds, or to see internal lights or visions during meditation or at night before going to sleep. In some cases, the subject seems to develop siddhi (powers) that appear to be in conflict with basic laws of the universe.

And then one day it happens. It is as though the body has accumulated so much energy that it can hold no more without bursting at the seams. And now, while the subject is resting or meditating, the rising of the accumulated energy takes place. In most cases, the surge is so powerful that the subject loses control and is at the mercy of the event. It is likely that he loses consciousness of his body while maintaining some sort of internal consciousness. During this period he experiences himself as a disembodied being of pure energy. Or perhaps he experiences profound bliss, or sees a magnificent, overwhelming vision of God—it is different for each subject.

Soon the excesses of energy within him abate and he comes down to earth. Whatever the experience was, he now knows that existence does not stop abruptly at the edges of the physical body. He was profoundly moved by the experience and will never be the same again.

Over the next few months, the Kundalini subject acclimates himself to the new world into which he has been thrust. There are many physiological changes to his body during this period, precipitated by the Kundalini awakening, itself. And there are more experiences to follow, although perhaps none as completely overwhelming as the classical awakening. But not only are there physiological changes to adapt to: the subject's attitudes toward the world around him are also thrown into a state of flux by the Kundalini event. It is a rebirth.

The remainder of this chapter describes the Kundalini subject's view of the time immediately preceding and following the Kundalini event. The material was prepared largely by abstracting and generalizing material from my own experiences as well as from the experiences of other Kundalini subjects. Unfortunately, as a Kundalini subject, I have formed opinions that may seem subjective to some readers. For the most part, I have tried to keep opinion, rationalization, and conjecture to myself, documenting only the perceptions of the Kundalini subject. However, where I felt it absolutely necessary to post an opinion, or to describe how Kundalini experts would justify certain experiences, I did so.

Physiological Effects

Many people believe that ESP phenomena are gifts to them from the blue. That is, they believe that seeing a vision clairvoyantly or precognitively is like watching a television set: nothing is demanded of the body in return for watching the picture.

One of the first things the Kundalini subject learns is that every gift exacts its demands of the body. Both the brain and the central nervous system seem to be involved in psychic sensing. But not only are these systems **affected** by psychic events, they are **modified** by them. Every transaction handled under the new world rules costs something, biologically speaking. And the effect on the body can be mild or severe, according to the intensity of the psychic event manifested in the subject. The subject will experience a wide range of effects from bliss, to headaches, to nervous irritations, welts on the body, temporary paralysis, temporary blindness, or other even more severe effects.

Teachers of Kundalini yoga say that these bodily effects are resistances—blocks, and impurities that are being burned away by the Kundalini fires. Likely, they are correct: it is probably the points of most resistance in the brain and central nervous system that are being burned by the excessive currents in these systems. This view is supported by the fact that the Kundalini subject will notice less of a demand on his body after a period of time.

There will be other physiological effects, too, such as internal visions, lights, and sounds, and strange movements of the body during meditation sessions. All of these correspond to activity in the brain and central nervous system.

Bliss: I once read somewhere that an itch is really a low-grade pain. It is likely that the physical bliss noticed by the Kundalini subject (and by heavy meditators) is a low-grade irritation of portions of the brain and central nervous system. Such bliss can be caused by meditating for a prolonged period or by generating alpha or theta waves on a biofeedback machine.* Usually, this bliss will continue for some time after meditation has ceased. It is almost as though one has exercised "muscles in the brain" that one has not used for some time. Over a period of months, the brain will seem to get used to these states and the bliss will not be as pronounced as it was near the time of the Kundalini event.

Bliss, like pleasure, comes in many degrees. It can range from a simple physical bliss, like the feeling you sometimes notice when you awaken in that pleasant, groggy state in the middle of the night, to a profound feeling of well-being, joy, and oneness with everything.

Heat and Pressure: Constant meditation and the resultant build-up of electrical energy within the body is sometimes felt as heat, pressure, and light (the last of which will be discussed separately). These effects are most noticeable in the diaphragm, back, neck, and head. Again, the effect occurs at a place where there is a blockage, or resistance, to the electrical activity.

Perhaps the most interesting area in which heat and pressure are felt is the head. The effect might be localized at one or more specific points, or it might be felt more generally over the entire head. When occurring in light doses, the effect can be very pleasurable. And when prolonged, light stupor or residual bliss result. But when it occurs in heavier amounts, the effect becomes painful and unpleasant. Luckily, the Kundalini subject has some control over whether this experience takes place, and to what degree.

Soon the Kundalini subject attains a high degree of control over the effect. He may be able to select specific spots to be heated, some seemingly as small as a dime.

The Kundalini subject notices other effects, too. He may feel an itching sensation on his cheeks, arms, or back during

---

*Refer to Appendix A for a discussion of brainwave states and biofeedback techniques.

meditation sessions. Or he may feel his eyelids jump, as though some external object had brushed lightly against them. When resting, or just as he enters his meditation sessions, he may have the sensation that the hair on his arms or legs is standing on end.

Pain: Some of the effects of the Kundalini event are as obvious to the subject as running into a wall. Pain is one of these. As you might expect, the subject will react adversely to these unenjoyable experiences, even going so far as to alter his spiritual disciplines to try to prevent their recurrence or to cut down on their intensity. Sometimes he will find himself stuck in the middle, beckoning to Kundalini with one hand and warding her off with the other.

The subject may experience sharp pains in the head, torso, arms, or legs. Or he may experience specific nerve bundle reactions, not unlike painful shingles, in which red blotches appear on his back, arms, or chest. Pains in the chest can be particularly frightening.

As a general rule, any pain that occurs in an area where other effects, such as bliss, heat, or pressure have been noticed previously is probably Kundalini-related.

Yogic Illnesses: It is now known that excessive and prolonged stress will bring various illnesses to the body. These illnesses are recorded in the person's muscle and tissue structures over a period of time prior to the actual manifestation of the disease.

Meditation will unstress some of these grooved structures. In unstressing in this manner, the meditator removes the impurities that will eventually cause the disease to manifest if stress is otherwise permitted to accumulate.

While these potential illnesses are being undone, or played out at an accelerated rate, the subject will experience symptoms of the disease to which he is prone. And so, stomach problems, heart palpitations, headaches, colds, and other manifestations will become more severe for a period of time.

In some cases, even though the illnesses are being "exorcised" from his body, this effect can be dangerous. For example, if the subject has inherent heart problems, it is conceivable that he could die from the increased activity. (The coroner's report here would have to be given as "Death due to accelerated healing.") It is reasonable, therefore, that people with heart problems or other serious disorders of the body or mind should shy away from the Kundalini experience and from **excessive** meditation.*

Of course, Kundalini subjects would argue that the risk is worth it because dying without having known your self is like never having lived at all.

Visions, Lights, and Sounds: Immediately preceding the Kundalini event, the subject will notice an increase in the number and intensity of visions he experiences during meditation sessions or quiet times. These images will seem to spring upon him from nowhere. He may see complex geometric structures or visions of simple, mundane items such as weeds, sticks, fields of flowers, doorstops, paperweights, or other such objects. Or he may see faces, other's or his own, or spiritual subjects, still or moving. Almost any picture may blossom to life within him.

Some of the subject's visions are simple hallucinations. That is, they are visions that spring from stored memories within the subject, and they have no feeling of being anything other than a perceived image. But there is another class of images that are much more vital. These images are **felt** and **experienced** as an actual environment in which part of the subject's consciousness now seems to operate. Perhaps some aspect of the subject's being has been transported to these places, or perhaps he has become conscious in these places while his physical body remains meditating in the chair or bed. I have dubbed these images **feelies** because of the very real presence felt during these events. Feelies are very exciting because they seem to bring two realities together at the same point in the here and now. Their workings will be covered in detail in part 2.

Visions, like bliss, heat and pressure, begin to fade and diminish in number with time.

In addition to his visions, the Kundalini subject experiences many different kinds of internal lights, sounds, and thoughts

---

*A number of Kundalini subjects, and I give as an example, Franklin Jones, have suffered unstressing attacks that mimicked painful and frightening heart failures. Kundalini is truely no game for the weak at heart. Refer to *"The Knee of Listening,"* by Franklin Jones, published by the Dawn Horse Press, for details of the symptoms Franklin experienced.

occurring at various intensities. At times the subject may notice a harsh white light flickering at about a four-to-seven cycle rate behind closed eyes. Or he may become filled with a soft white light that lacks the harsh definition of the flickering light. Sometimes the subject will see white light rolling and washing around like waves at the seashore. At other times, the lights will take on a blue or purple color and will wax and wane, each pulse advancing into nothingness after the previous one.

From time to time, another form of light will appear. These are miniature suns, little pinpricks of intensely bright light against the black field of vision behind closed eyelids. These lights flicker into being and then disappear in rapid order. The subject cannot predict where these individual miniature suns will make their appearance. That is, their positions are not fixed.

A slightly modified form of this effect is called *chinmay*. With the *chinmay* effect, the image begins to break up, evaporate, as though all of the solidity in the object being perceived has been drawn off into the void. The world is resolved, temporarily, as a host of small, rapidly moving pinpricks. Usually this effect is most noticeable when the subject looks at an expansive, solid field such as a wall, rug, or perhaps the sky. It is similar to the effect of the moving phosphenes one normally sees when looking at the blue sky, only much more pronounced.

The coming of the Kundalini event may be signaled by dreams in which a large, bright sun, or other bright lights, such as the headlights of a car, are seen. As the Kundalini event gets closer these dream lights will become prominent in meditation sessions as well as in dreams. That is, during meditation, the subject will catch a quick glimpse of the rising or setting sun, or he will imagine he has seen a bright light reflecting off a mirror. This event indicates that an electrical path within the brain is becoming stimulated by excessive electrical currents associated with the Kundalini. In mystic terminology, the "third eye" is being readied to be opened.

After the Kundalini event has taken place, the subject may be able to see the sun while going about his daily affairs. At times, he may also be able to see a bright blue spot in the position normally reserved for the sun, while at other times there may be only a dark spot there, like a blind spot.

The subject may develop a visual sensitivity to a certain shade of blue. Sometimes a blue spot will be projected outward onto the white pages of a book or newspaper. After a few months this effect will taper off. However, each time thereafter that the Kundalini currents build up, the subject will again notice the sun and the blue spot.

The experience of light is usually pleasant. However, in some cases the light can be extremely bright, surpassing (subjectively) even the brightness of the sun. The Biblical Paul, for instance, was blinded on the road to Damascus and remained without vision for three days.

The Kundalini subject will also notice many sounds during meditative and quiet periods. He will hear a plethora of chirps, clicks, knocks, whistles, roaring or rushing sounds, and other "science fiction" sound effects.

He will also hear thoughts whose origins appear to be from deep within, but the contexts of which seem to be nonsensical and out of place. To some subjects, these inner thoughts become quite strong and disruptive even during the performance of daily routines. Someone who has never attempted to trace the origin and "route" of his own thoughts might easily come to believe that "other" voices are talking to him in his head, or that God or the Devil is asking him to behave in one fashion or another.

Of course, some of these thoughts may actually **be** the thoughts of other beings. The frightening thing about this, until one gets used to it, is that one can't really tell whether a particular thought originates within him or comes from some external source—the thought is just there, without any flags or names to identify its true origin. After a period of time, the idea of not being able to say "mine" or "not-mine" to each thought that springs up becomes less of a concern to the Kundalini subject. In fact, this knowledge helps to open him up, dissolve his ego, remove his limitations, and give him some freedom for the first time in his life.

Kriyas: *Kriyas* are spontaneous body movements or mental activities that take place during meditation or when the subject is otherwise resting. They are caused by an internal discharge of accumulated energy that manifests in a movement of the body or mind. Because they are not directly controlled by the conscious intellect, they can be frightening to the person who is not familiar with them.

Kriyas take many forms. They can range from simple muscle twitching, similar to that experienced by most of us sometimes in our lives, to wild thrashing or shaking movements of the body that can continue for minutes.

Sometimes the *Kriyas* take the form of *"Mudra,"* or dance-like hand and body positions. The yogis practice various *asanas* (postures) in their yoga classes to make it easier for the body to assume these positions when called upon to do so.

For some subjects, *Kriyas* can take the form of roaring, barking, whistling, laughing, crying, or screaming sounds. They can be awesome to behold.

Although *Kriyas* can be frightening at first, they are never really out of control because they can quickly be turned off by the conscious intellect. And this is usually what happens the first few times they occur.

Kundalini teachers believe that *Kriyas,* like other physiological manifestations, are simply indicative of one's impurities being burned out by the Kundalini energies. And indeed, like the other physiological manifestations, they usually die down and disappear a few months after they first appear.

Kriyas are almost always blissful. While they are occurring, and afterward, the body is permeated with euphoria and a sense of well-being. Apparently *Kriyas,* like yogic illnesses, are another, more immediate, form of the unstressing phenomenon. It is as though the internal knots and illnesses that have been with the subject all his life are suddenly and briskly undone. And now he simply wants to remain sitting, basking in the newfound peace within him.

Some *Kriyas* can be experienced subtly, without concurrent body movements. For example, the meditator might experience an inner mental episode in which his thoughts are caught up in a repetitive "movement," while his outer body remains still. In such a case, a swishing of electricity in his head may be converted into an inner voice repeating a certain syllable over and over again. After such an occurrence, the subject understands how *Kriyas* happen: he sees that if there was just a little more power behind the electrical event, or if the electrical discharge occurred at another spot in the brain, his physical body would have moved, just as his inner thoughts had moved.

While all of the effects in this chapter are physiological in origin, the ones covered to this point are the more immediate, obvious ones. The remainder of this chapter is devoted to some of the longer term effects and attitudinal changes in the Kundalini subject.

Spiritual Weightlessness

Those of you who have had the opportunity to lose large amounts of weight over a short period of time, or those of you who have fasted, will understand the feeling of spiritual weightlessness: the rest may find it a bit more difficult to comprehend.

Around the time of the Kundalini awakening, the subject will begin to notice a feeling of buoyancy, lightness of attitude, lightness of mind and body. This can cause him to develop giggling spells or to pun incessantly. It is as though a part of his being has been banished from the basic being, thereby making him "lighter." In some instances, the subject may get the impression that part of him is "hanging around the outside somewhere," waiting to get back in. (Perhaps the Kundalini currents have rearranged the relationship between the right and left hemispheres of the brain, leaving him partly bicameral.)

During this period, the Kundalini subject, his family, and his close friends may experience a number of mysterious electrical phenomena. For example, they may feel the unseen touches of a ghostly hand, or they may feel as though they have run into a spider web when none is there, and so on. One might speculate that part of the subject *has* been relegated to the "outside," wherever that may be.

While in this stage, the subject is likely to be more compassionate and loving (non-sexual) than he was previously. Anger and fear may have largely disappeared from his repertoire of emotions.

Over a period of months, the feeling of weightlessness may give way to a filling in of the former weight. Anger and other strong emotions may return. It is possible that this reintegration will come rapidly and forcefully, in which case the subject may temporarily feel as though he has been possessed.

Celibacy and Other Austerities

Earlier the concept of "putting the cart before the horse" was mentioned in the context of eager, but naive, Kundalini hopefuls practicing all sorts of austerities such as the elimination of sex, renunciation of worldly possessions, and other self-imposed tortures. The person who has been struck by Kundalini will come naturally to some of these austerities after the awakening.

There will be periods ranging into the months, perhaps longer, in which he will not desire sex. In fact, there are some short periods in which sex will be "penalized" by severe nausea and sharp pain in the sex organs. Under these conditions, one learns quickly when to abstain.

During these periods, lust will have melted away. There will be no eye for the other sex. However, natural functions will return at a later date. Note that the period in which sex is rejected is not a hardship for the Kundalini subject. (I can't, however, speak for his or her spouse.)

Other negative practices will also fall away of their own accord, even if they were previously deeply ingrained in the subject. For example, the desire for alcohol may disappear. In some cases, the body will develop an intolerance for it. The need for cigarettes may also drop. Soon, the subject may notice that he is developing an aversion to some of the heavier meats such as pork and rare beef. He may become a vegetarian.

Again, these stages are temporary. The subject's body will let him know what it needs and what it doesn't need.

Emotional and Attitudinal Changes

We have all had days in which we carry over attitudes and emotions from one situation into the next. For example, if you have a particularly disagreeable day at work, it is possible that you might be short with your family when you get home. In fact, when you examine your reaction to daily situations closely, you see that you tend to carry over your feelings and biases, positive and negative, in almost all of your transactions with the outside world.

The Hindus refer to this carrying over of emotion and

attitude as *karma:* pattern formed through ignorance. According to the Hindus, *karma* prevents us from seeing events as they really are. Further, the *karma* formation becomes habitual, and we begin to accumulate *karma* through our individual tendencies toward guilt, anger, anxiety, unforgivingness, and other negative traits. This, according to the Hindus, prevents one from experiencing enlightenment, and must all be played out, or exhausted, before one can know one's self.

Karma can be undone naturally, and further formation prevented, by practicing meditation. For this reason, the emotional and attitudinal changes noted by the Kundalini subject are experienced to a degree by all who practice meditation.

The meditator soon notices that there are fewer and fewer events that are life or death affairs. He finds that he has no need either to express or to repress strong negative emotions because they just aren't there any longer.

As the subject watches the *karma-forming* mechanism disappear, he finds himself relaxing—perhaps for the first time ever. He begins to have fun in his relationships with others. He becomes more truthful in his dealings because he has no set programs to defend. He begins to live in the here and now without worrying about his past or future activity.

But paradoxically, at the same time as the subject's *karma-forming* mechanism begins to disappear, a new form of *karma* begins to surface: the subject feels a growing disenchantment with all of the "wrong" situations in his life. For example, if he did not follow his natural leanings in selecting a career, if he was diverted by the thought of making more money or working with a friend, he now becomes disenchanted with his work. The things that have become wrong for him are now like thorns in his foot, and he soon acts to correct these situations.

This may mean that he gives up a $30,000 job to sell home-grown vegetables along the side of a country road; it may mean that he abandons family and friends to become a nomad, traveling aimlessly from place to place; or it may mean that he gives up his vagabond ways to become a man of the cloth or a respected businessman.

Temporarily, for as long as it takes him to right his ways, the Kundalini subject will undergo increased suffering at the hands of his disenchantment. This is because his love for money and other false images, which has become habitual, is now in conflict with his newfound sense of right values. And so, a war between right thinking and false goals is fought within him.

Eventually right thinking wins: the desire for money turns sour and convenience relationships lose their convenience, vividly displaying what remains.

Unfortunately, disenchantment, even with the "wrong" things in life, is still a form of *karma*. This, too, must go before the final realization of self can take place.

Changed Dream Content

Hundreds of books have been written and much has been learned about all aspects of dreams. And indeed, dreams deserve such extensive treatment: they are highly complex affairs and are probably an integral part of nature's way to maintain and balance the human in his environment.

It seems that innumerable components go into the production of each dream. At times, simple external stimuli, such as light shining through a crack in the window shade, seem to be translated into dream components; at other times, body conditions—for example, an upset stomach, or an arm that is asleep—can influence the dream content.

Dreams can play out desires that are otherwise repressed. They can fulfill wishes; they can vividly portray the things that are bothering the dreamer in waking life.

And then there are the more esoteric functions that dreams seem to play: they can sometimes outline events to come, or seemingly carry some aspect of the dreamer's being to other places or times. Occasionally, the dreamer seems to be telepathic. And sometimes it even seems that external entities use the dream medium as a vehicle for communicating directly with the dreamer.

Dreams seem to function as "community bulletin boards," informing all aspects of the dreamer about what concerns him.

Most teachers of the various esoteric yogas claim that dreaming ceases, or is reduced greatly, after the dreamer attains enlightenment. If this is true, the concept that dreams are part of a balancing mechanism—keeping the dreamer in tune with himself and the universe — makes sense, since the enlightened being is supposedly in tune and would not need to dream.

In any case, just prior to the Kundalini event, and for a number of months after, the subject's dream content changes drastically. The dreams cover a broader scope than before. They describe a larger, more diverse existence. It appears that the dreams attempt to balance the dreamer in a more expansive environment than before. One indication of this is that the subject will notice a preponderance of dreams that he is unable to interpret using his historical dream symbology: he is forced to update his unique library of personal symbols.

In his waking life, the Kundalini subject is more aware of his internal functions than he was before. In addition, he is undergoing a number of physiological changes that manifest as psychic events. All of these effects are reflected in his dream world. The subject will notice a higher incidence of precognitive and telepathic dreams. He will also note many dream series over a period of weeks or months, that reflect the status of the internal changes he is undergoing.

Around the time of the Kundalini event itself, he will probably have dreams that reflect the increased electrical currents within his brain. These dreams can take the form of rising water, tornados, electrical storms, and the like. The subject may also have dreams symbolizing attainment or death.

In "Spiritual Weightlessness" I explained the feeling the Kundalini subject has that portions of his being have been banished, and are hovering about "outside" somewhere. This, too, is reflected in his dream world. The subject will be tempted in his dreams by the banished functions. That is, surrogate animus or anima symbols will proposition the subject to regain entry, or reassimilate, into the total psyche. Or the dreams may be less specific, with the banished functions being represented simply by darkness — the "black."

In my opinion, Christ's temptation in the wilderness was such a phenomenon. In his case, however, the Kundalini experience was so devastating that the subliminal activity broke into his waking consciousness.

The subject who is not familiar with this phenomenon may suspect that he is going crazy, or that demons are attempting to possess him.

Awareness of the Internal/External Servomechanism

"Do unto others as you would have them do unto you."

This mystic saying does more than just ensure nice treatment at the hands of others. Its meaning is rooted in the way each man directs the creation and maintenance of his body and mind. The Kundalini subject soon learns that how he deals with the external world determines how he deals with himself, and vice versa.

In addition to his external consciousness, man also possesses an internal, or biological consciousness. While the external consciousness takes care of surface functions such as conceptualizing, perceiving, sensing and rationalizing, the internal consciousness controls growth, removes poisons from the body, creates the sperm, moves the infection-fighting cells to the wound, digests the food, and directs many other thankless, "unconscious" functions.

Together, these internal and external systems form a single, servomechanistic command system to ensure man's survival in a changing environment. The internal consciousness ensures the basic, "intra-survival" of man, while the external consciousness helps man survive in the external world. Total survival demands that they work together.

While the internal consciousness knows only survival, the external system is slightly different. Apparently, somewhere along man's evolutionary path man's external control system went askew. Not only does it now concern itself with survival, but it allows itself to be distracted by toys, frustrations, unfounded anxieties, sins, social laws, and other weird concepts that don't directly deal with the organism's survival.

And of course these concepts are totally alien to the inner, biological system. Nevertheless, it must go on performing according to the instructions it receives from the external world. It must interpret these confusing stimuli to regulate the heart, fight the infection, digest the food, and control all other internal activities.

Likewise, man's perception of the external world is colored by the way he feels within. Internal confusion and disease will cause him to see reflections of these in the external world: perplexity, confusion, chaos, destruction, evil, and sin will be projected outward and superimposed on his environment.

In a normal man, there is quite a gap between the internal and external systems. The servomechanism is slow, but forgiving, and it takes quite a few conscious, negative instructions before the biological system will begin to go wrong. Not so for the Kundalini subject. The gap shortens for him! His internal systems will quickly react to his emotions and thoughts. If these are negative or confusing, he will quickly bring disease to his system; if they are positive and clear, he will be at peace within. This is a natural failsafe mechanism that ensures that a man of knowledge will be beneficial, rather than destructive, to others. For if he harms others, he harms himself.

The gap lessens each day. Soon, what is thought, **is.** Soon the slightest negative thought brings digestive disruptions and other negative physiological disturbances, while when things are right in the external world, things are right within.

It is not difficult to see why the Kundalini aspirant should work on making himself a better person: it is for his own protection, and not because some do-good moralist has proclaimed that he must be a good person before God will give him the gift!

The Satsang Effect

The Hindus believe that one of the most efficient ways to become a self-realized being is to associate closely with one who is already self-realized: to sit quietly with him in *Satsang*, absorbing his radiance. The idea is that by sitting in such a being's presence, the seeker of self will become like him.

Itzhak Bentov, in *"Stalking the Wild Pendulum,"* refers to a well-known physical effect called "rhythm entrainment," which illustrates how the *satsang* mechanism might work. In Bentov's example of this effect, a number of identical grandfather clocks are lined against a wall and started with pendulums at different positions. In a relatively short time, the pendulums all move synchronously.

A similar effect is exhibited when you strike a tuning fork near others of its kind. Tuning forks having the same, or nearly the same, oscillating frequency will vibrate and hum as though they were the ones that had been struck.

From these examples, it should not be difficult to see the

plausability of such an effect happening with living beings.
And such is the case: the pre-Kundalini subject senses a
certain excitement about the presence of a self-realized being
or a being in whom the Kundalini energies are active. Such
a one will seem to ebb and flow with an energy that can't
quite be seen, but that seems to shimmer about him at times
modifying the outlines of his body. His movements seem
effortless; at times he appears almost to float from place to
place. He crackles with an undefinable vitality. Yet there
is a silence, a peacefulness, a natural serenity about him.
The pre-Kundalini subject soon begins to absorb and manifest
these highly contagious qualities himself.

One who has been struck by the Kundalini will notice
that the level of his own vitality will affect others around him.
In his silence, they will be silent; when he is emotion-filled,
they will be emotion-filled; when he experiences high levels
of psychic activity, they too will manifest psychic events.
His close friends will report out-of-body experiences, lucid
dreams, electrical phenomena, visions, internal lights, and
similar experiences.

Traveling in the company of other spiritual or psychic
seekers is one of the most important things the Kundalini
subject, or aspirant, can do: it provides positive reinforcement
from other people that these experiences are not merely
individual hallucinations. *Satsang* will alter the participant's
beliefs about what our agreed-upon reality permits in the way
of daily experience of life.

Concept and Paradox Resolution

Mystic parlance is studded with paradoxical declarations
that pit the absolute against the relative. For example:

- As we know more about the universe, we know less.
- The man who knows all is the man who knows nothing.
- To live, you must first die.

From the standpoint of the logical, rational intellect, which
must always remain in a relative reality, these paradoxes
cannot be resolved. None can fathom, with rational mind, the

extent of eternity; none can find the "smallest" particle or the most distant star. There is always something smaller, something larger, something farther out or farther in. The rational mind cannot decide whether something exists outside of "everything," or whether everything is everything: both thoughts are unfathomable.

Nevertheless, a strange thing happens to the Kundalini subject: he finds that he can resolve more and more of the paradoxes that previously plagued him. He is able to resolve them because, for short periods of time, he sees them from the viewpoint of God, rather than man. He stands outside and above himself, so to speak, to see how things really are. He becomes part of the absolute reality, rather than a relative reality. And he sees that from this view, there are no paradoxes.

But these moments are fleeting. And when they go, they leave only a lingering scent in the rational mind. And now, when the Kundalini subject tries to explain his newfound knowledge, he again becomes man. His sense of accomplishment, his pride, his rational mind trying to categorize the events that have taken place—all of these bring him back to earth. So now his tongue clucks and his teeth tie up. The futility of this situation causes frustration to rise up in him, and soon he learns to be silent.

As the Kundalini subject understands more deeply that there are no paradoxes, they lose their vitality in his life. The burning will to solve, intellectually, the whys and wherefores of the universe begin to evaporate in the light of intuition. And this intuitive knowledge that now shines through him fosters an environment in which *just being* becomes his life's vitality.

One might expect that the Kundalini subject, believing that man's concepts are but illusions, would reject conceptual thinking and balk at living within today's societal structures. While this can happen, it is not necessarily the case: being aware of the illusion does not of itself cause man to reject the world or his God-given abilities. In fact, the Kundalini life force amplifies the subject's waking intellect so that he can function more creatively in his daily routines. The Kundalini subject continues to use man's concepts to survive and to bring others, when they ask, to the point where they can begin to uncover their own truths.

Event Control

To this point, the view of the Kundalini subject can be largely explained under the normally accepted laws of time and space. The remainder of this chapter deals with perceptions that are more difficult to explain under the existing laws of reality. Nevertheless, they are certainly valid perceptions of the Kundalini subject — they belong to his world — and they deserve coverage here.

"Event control" is such a perception. The Kundalini subject notices a new willingness of the world to cooperate with his wants. He becomes a sorcerer, of sorts. Business meetings turn out according to his wishes; people whom he wants to like him do so; events seem to fall into place magically. And what he needs in work and in private life always seems to be provided for him. He does not know how these things come about, they just seem to happen.

The Kundalini subject develops a sense of responsibility to keep other people from being adversely affected by his newfound ability. He learns this responsibility rather quickly, as there seems to be a universal law of reflection that returns the fruits of ill wishes to the ill-wisher. This is another of the many reasons why the Kundalini seeker should strive constantly to better himself through love and right action.

Control of the Force

One day while Carl Jung was speaking with Sigmund Freud on psychic phenomena, he noticed a band of heat building up around his midsection. This was followed shortly by a loud explosion (which damaged nothing) from the bookcase near which they stood. Subsequently, a second clap came, after which the heat in Jung's stomach subsided. No more strange explosions were noted after this.

It is likely that the above was a weak manifestation of the poltergeist effect, where things are mysteriously lifted by some unseen force and flung about the room recklessly.

This mysterious effect may also be noticed by the Kundalini subject. During certain periods of deep meditation, for example, he may be startled to hear the wall crack loudly next to him. Or he may see the lights flicker on and off for no apparent reason.

While at first the subject may intellectually question that he is somehow related to these mysterious events, he will come to recognize over a period of time that they **do** follow his internal electrical states. When he is quiet internally, things will be quiet externally; when he is agitated, things will be restless in the outer world. He will soon come to believe that he is indeed related to these events in some unknown way.

Apparently, he unconsciously controls some sort of force that is not normally gathered in sufficient strength or quantity to cause these effects. It is feasible, although I personally have seen no evidence to substantiate this, that levitation (lifting one's self from the ground with no visible means), psychokinesis (moving objects with the mind), and the occurrence of spontaneous fires and other "devilish" events are the result of such unconscious manipulation of this force.

Of course, there are many theories about how such an effect could take place. And all are equally valid, since we can now prove none of them. For example, the following is a note I made a few years ago about how the awakened man might maneuver in unusual fashion through a universe of infinite probabilities.

The unawakened man sees only envelopes of reality; he sees a filtered, minimum set of "most-likely" probabilities as dictated by his self-imposed limitations. In his universe, only a limited number of events is possible.

But the awakened man who pricks the bubble of illusion has no limiting factors to predetermine what he can or cannot see. He has no attitudes carved in stone, no fears of things to come, no guilt or worry about things past, no biased opinions toward or against anything he might perceive. Such a man sees the universe as a range of infinite probabilities and possibilities.

Perhaps it is possible for the awakened man to skip about through these probabilities as a water bug skips about on the surface of a lake. Perhaps such a man could temporarily disassociate himself from the "universal probability matrix" and then program his reentry into a less likely, but more interesting, set of circumstances.

Could this temporary disabling of his relative existence put him beyond time and space, if but for a frac-

tion of a second? And could this be the mechanism for "seeing out of time," or for moving objects with the mind, or for doing anything not currently in our individual or collective agreements on how we view reality?

If the awakened man could learn how to plot his coordinates for reentry into his relative existence, rather than falling slavishly into a most-likely probability, he would effectively create a new universe with each reentry. And so he could travel into an arrangement in which objects are displaced in space, or in which his body has mysteriously "traveled" from one location to another, or in which objects have been reshaped according to his whims. Or perhaps he might simply select a thought to be present in the mind of a friend. All kinds of delicious possibilities could be arranged at reentry.

And of course, to all others except the awakened one, the universe has really remained linear and relative throughout the whole magic act.

There is a popular theory that as more and more people meditate, and as more and more impurities are burned off into the external world, there will be a collective effect felt on the earth itself. In this theory, natural calamities will increase as the number of meditators and Kundalini subjects increases until the combined force is so strong that the heavens themselves will open.

Perhaps when Christ told the people that the time will come when no walls built by man will be left standing, he knew of this effect through his own experience, and he deduced that when more people lined themselves up on the side of spirituality and psychic manifestations, the material world would reap the havoc. Perhaps this is why he was able to predict signs of times that would herald cataclysmic events to follow.

The Total Effect

The Kundalini subject sees his concepts of self and reality shattered by the classical event. But even more earth shaking, in the long run, he must adapt to existence in the new world into which he has been thrust.

The Kundalini subject undergoes many physiological

changes and manifestations of these changes. He experiences new heights of bliss, joy, and other positive states, But he also sees his share of pain, trepidation, and disenchantment with certain choices of life style. He may undergo a number of frightening yogic illnesses. He experiences many pleasant visions, and some not so pleasant. He hears various sounds and voices. At times, his body seems to act on its own. He sees his negative emotions banished to some unreachable place in his psyche, and he follows their attempts to reintegrate. His intellect is upgraded while his value judgements about what is important to him change radically. He begins to experience oneness within his own body mechanisms.

The laws of time and space change also. The Kundalini subject experiences many unusual psychic effects that defy explanation. He affects the world around him in some unknown way. He seems to wield a strange, psychic force that is not yet under his full control. He finds that he not only knows what is happening at the present moment, but he can also sense shadows, or overtones, of what will be. It is as though the present point has expanded its boundaries forward and backward from the here and now.

The subject's rigid, linear, space-time walls have crumbled. He finds himself existing in a flux of space-time, rather than in a specific, rock-bound place in a time-locked moment.

All of this takes time to adapt to.

A SUMMARY OF PART ONE

The Kundalini event has been called many names by many different people of various beliefs across the ages. And today it lies buried within the tenets of many, if not all, of the exoteric religions.

In the esoteric, non-technical view, it is a spiritual or psychic event—a direct tie with God or self through personal experience.

However, the Western technologist, not recognizing the evolutionary aspect of Kundalini, sees it as a sickness to be cured; nervousness to be tranquilized; personality components to be integrated or destroyed.

But Kundalini events are on the increase in the West, precipitated perhaps by the hungry spiritual appetites spawned by materialism and its selfish, separatist concepts. And whether or not Kundalini is pathological, it is happening.

With the right attitude, you can survive it. In fact, it can be a blessing to those who are ready to accept it.

PART 2: KUNDALINI ME

PROLOGUE TO PART TWO

In *"Knee of Listening,"* published by Dawn Horse Press, Franklin Jones describes a feeling of light and vitality that occasionally permeated him when he was a child. He called this his "bright."

It was while I was reading about Franklin Jones' "bright" that I realized I, too, had a "bright" when I was a child. I first noticed it when I was about 12 years old, in seventh grade.

It was May Day, 1951, and Mr. Miller, our twinkley-eyed, white-haired, math teacher was hosting the annual Junior High, Rapid Calculation contest. This event was actually held for the benefit of the Commercial students, whose curriculum included rapid calculation and whose careers would take them into areas such as Certified Public Accounting, Banking, grocery store clerking, and so on. However, the contest was open to the Academic, college-bound students and to the General, blue-collar workers as well.

I was an Academic student with no training in rapid calculation, so I was one of those not expected to fare well in the contest. But I knew from previous experience that I was pretty good with numbers, and besides, no other contest that interested me was being held at this time of the day. So there I was.

As Mr. Miller began reading the first question, I could feel the excitement thrill through my entire body. I became hyper, vibrating physically with some inner energy that I had not experienced before. And I noticed a brightness through and about me — a light that had never been so bright before. In a way the feeling was similar to, but stronger than, the activity one feels in his midsection just before throwing up. But now it was noticeable throughout the whole body, and was a good feeling, an "alive" feeling, rather than a sensation of sickness.

Mr. Miller finished reading the first question, "— times a dozen and a half, minus 14, divided by four equals? — "

"Twenty-eight!" The answer was literally **thrown** out of my mouth by some forceful inner impulse. I couldn't have stopped it if I wanted to!

"That's right," he said, as he scanned my general area to

identify the person who had answered. "Who was that?"
I identified myself sheepishly.

"And how'd you get it?"

I thought about that for a second or two, and then told him
I didn't know. And it was to remain this way for the rest
of the contest and for the next four years of contests—I never
knew how I got the answers! I could feel them being worked
out, or at least I could feel some kind of super fast activity
going on within me, but I couldn't begin to track it consciously. I never really knew whether I was reading Mr. Miller's
mind as he looked at the answer sheet, or whether I was
somehow figuring out the answers internally, at super speed.

At the end of the regulation contest, I was tied with a
fellow named Claude Wambold. Mr. Miller took us into private chambers to finish the contest. I won it handily, as I
did two more times, plus one second place finish, over the
next four years.

However, as I approached 12th grade, my bright began to
show itself less and less during these contests. And by the
time I reached 12th grade it had disappeared nearly altogether. In that year, I was forced to compete under normal
circumstances and as a result was beaten soundly by a class-
mate named Neal Coyle and a number of others. I didn't
even place.

But I never forgot that feeling in my body in those exciting
times. I never forgot the feeling of racing my inner intellect
down the superhighway at top speed, burning the carbon
deposits out of my mental carburetor.

I was now about 23 years old. After High School I had
joined the Army to serve a hitch, and then I joined IBM,
where I worked as a Computer Field Engineer servicing an
air defense computer at Newburgh, New York. During this
period in my life, many strange psychic occurrences took
place. For example, one weekend, as I was driving to Pennsylvania to visit my family, I began to feel very queasy behind
the wheel. This feeling of uneasiness rapidly intensified,
leaving me feeling extremely weak and "washed out," and
finally, almost unable to move my body. It was as though I had
gone into shock. I mustered all of my remaining strength and
pulled over to the side of the road, at which time nearly all of
my consciousness seemed to leave my body. I felt literally like

a block of wood, drained of all the "stuff"that makes me go.

I sat there, unable to move for a few minutes. Then, very slowly, my faculties began to return to me. At this time my body began to shake and flutter, as from extreme nervousness. Finally, I got control of myself and pulled back onto the road. I rounded the corner slowly and saw a gruesome sight. There, only about three hundred yards or so from where I had stopped, was a serious accident involving two cars. By the time I got there, a number of other cars had stopped, and I was waved through. But I knew that the accident had happened around the time that I began to feel so strange. I have since often wondered whether I would have been involved in that accident, had I continued without stopping (and whether some Guardian Angel had warned me off), or whether I had felt, through empathy, the emotions of one or more of the people involved in the accident. I suppose I will never know.

At about this time, I discovered that I had a telepathic link with my sister, Sue. It seemed that many of my dreams directly reflected something she was reading, thinking, or talking about. I soon got into the habit of calling home every time I had an unusual dream to find out what she was thinking or doing at that moment. (Because I was a shift worker, this was a reasonable thing to do, as it didn't disturb her sleep.)

I started recording and interpreting my dreams after I experienced a very strong, "lucid" dream that turned out to be telepathic, as well. The dream occurred at about 2:00 on a Saturday on which I had not made the trip home to Pennsylvania. It was a normal, uneventful dream until a fuzzy image flitted into view. The fact that I couldn't focus on it caused me to realize that I was dreaming. With this knowledge came the realization that I had full control over my dream, and should be able to "force" the image into focus. At once, a clear picture of footprints on a printed page blossomed into view. The footprints were indicating a trail from place to place, stopping and changing direction at each item pictured on the page. The last item they came to sprang into full view with a startling intensity. It was a commode with a long, green hand coming up out of the bowl. I was overcome with a feeling of revulsion and awakened.

The next weekend I traveled to Pennsylvania, where I

discovered that my sister had just received in the mail a small novelty commode with a cute verse written on it. When the lid was lifted, a green hand would snake out of the bowl. This, of course, reminded me of the dream I had the week before. I questioned Sue about it, and she was able to remember, because of a television show she was watching concurrently, that at 2:00 o'clock on that Saturday she was looking at a catalog of novelty items. She was wondering when the novelty she had ordered (the commode) would arrive in the mail, as she had sent for it some time before. She had looked at the bowl and was temporarily struck with a feeling of revulsion.

I began to purchase books on all aspects of psychic phenomena, dream interpretation, and various esoteric and exoteric religions. These books seemed to open my belief structures thereby permitting the psychic experiences to build in intensity and frequency. But the more of these events I experienced, the more I began to shy away from them. I was in awe of these experiences, and fearful of the tremendous power they displayed. I was afraid I would be blown away.

Finally, shortly after I learned that my father was dying of cancer, I stopped reading my books and made every attempt to deny these experiences.

I was home in Pennsylvania in the bathroom one weekend. My legs had gone to sleep from sitting. When I got up to leave, a feeling of panic seemed to spread the tingling in my legs into my upper body. Soon it seemed that my entire body was vibrating furiously. I went out into the living room, panic running through me. I didn't know what was happening to me, and I was losing control. My mother asked me what was wrong. I told her "Nothing," and raced out of the house. I had to get some air.

Outside, it was dark and starry. The smell of wet grass was strong, but welcome, as my body continued to hum fiercely. I threw myself down on the ground, face-first into the grass, where I lay without moving, my arms spread to grab as much ground as they could.

My mother had followed me out, and again she asked what was wrong. Somehow I assured her that I would be all right, and convinced her to go back inside. Soon the vibrations began to play themselves out. The ground felt very, very good. I was able now to think about how my whole inner foundation had been wiped away, and how I had completely lost control of myself. I imagined that this is how earthquake victims must feel.

The whole incident was probably some sort of nervous collapse caused by the pressures of maintaining the family financially. Nevertheless, this event, with the concern caused by my father's condition, was sufficient to make me turn my back on things psychic "for good." Strangely enough, although I packed up my books, I didn't give them away or destroy them.

Twelve years later and I am 35, almost 36. I've been married for about 10 years, to a fine woman and understanding keeper, I might add. I've got two handsome boys, age five and four, and I work as a Technical Writer for IBM in Poughkeepsie, New York.

In the course of my duties, I meet a very intense, intelligent co-worker of German descent who is deeply interested in things psychic. So I get out my books again.

THE SETUP

Initially, I got off to a rough start in the Programming Technical Writing group. I had come from a field environment where job responsibilities were spread across a number of people, to the development laboratory, where responsibility was an individual affair. I had seven years experience as a Field Engineer, but little experience as a programmer, and no experience as a writer. Further, I had not attended college, so my command of the English language and my deportment in the professional business world were spotty, at best.

But I was a hard worker, and very competitive. And before too long, the pendulum had swung in the other direction for me: nothing could go wrong. As a result, I climbed quickly through the ranks, advancing from Junior Technician to Advisory Planner, a position which I hold today.

Through all of this, the projects came and were conquered, one by one. Nothing seemed to be insurmountable. And over the seven-year period from 1965 until 1972 I transformed myself from scapegoat into sacred cow. My peers respected my opinion and came to me often for advice.

Soon, however, I became conditioned to success. There was no longer any room for failure — it was unthinkable. I became walled-in by my own abilities. Instead of being my adornments, my talents and successes became my bonds, my jailers. My credo of "I must do it better than before" imprisoned me.

And then it happened. In 1972 I began to work on a project in which nothing was destined to go right. I had always been a nervous person, but now I got even worse. As things began to fall apart, I began to bare my teeth to my peers. Soon I found myself yelling in anger over the telephone and shouting people down in meetings. I was very frustrated, to say the least.

My smoking and drinking became a problem. I soon found myself smoking four packs of cigarettes a day. Sometimes I'd have two, or even three, of the filthy weeds going at once. And then I'd go home after a bad day at work and glug down half a fifth of Jack Daniels and a six-pack of beer before stumbling off to bed.

It soon became difficult for me to maintain my intensity at work without feeling some kind of discomfort. If I'd get into a heated discussion with one of my peers, my heart would begin to palpitate loudly and forcefully. I developed a chronic case of heartburn and I began to carry Rolaids, Aspirin, Librium and other temporary "cures" in my briefcase, which soon became more medicine bag than briefcase.

In 1974 things came to a head. By now I had spent the last two years generating an 8-inch stack of documents and memos, all of which were next to useless during this trying period. I became extremely impatient with my peers. When questions would arise, I would give the "right solution" without offering to explain why I felt that particular solution to be right. When someone would question my solution, I would show annoyance and say "Because that's the way it is," or some such answer. This usually terminated the event.

But then a new kid named Paul Myslenski moved on the block. Paul was an intelligent, gaunt, inquisitive fellow, an ex-teacher, who wouldn't take guff from anyone—even a sacred cow. I suppose I sensed this from the first day I met him. He would question everything. And he had soulful, piercing eyes that would stare through you if he didn't understand something you said. He made me very uncomfortable.

As I dealt with him on a continuing daily basis, I could feel my protective walls of superiority through time-in-service crumbling. The "institution," the franchise, was being riddled by this hungry, fresh kid's unwillingness to take a back seat.

What was worse, I could see that other people were beginning to question my superiority after watching Paul. They began to emulate his inquisitiveness and "show me" attitude. I suppose what I disliked most about him was that I saw a ghost of Tom Wolfe past. It was very much like looking into a mirror at the way I was six or eight years before: a success story in the making. And frankly, I was jealous.

One day Paul began his inquisitive nagging at something I had blessed as truth. I shouted my stock "Because that's how it is," and hoped that would end it. I was mad.

But his eyes deepened in anger and he got red in the face as he shouted, "Who the hell do you think you are? Are you the only one entitled to the truth?—You don't know a damned thing!

It was as though I had just taken a dive into a cold pool

of water. It was something my vast experience couldn't stand up to—a personal, philosophical attack. And something broke within me in that moment. I didn't have any reply, but now I didn't need one. Something had been released and was now floating freely in the air around us.

"*What am I doing?*" I thought. "*How did I get here?*" I reasoned that with much more of this, I would probably die of a heart attack soon. I could see the epitaph on my tombstone:

HERE LIES TOM WOLFE, THE INSTITUTION.
HE DIED SLUMPED OVER HIS DESK,
WHILE ARGUING WITH A NEW-HIRE.

The house of cards had finally come down, and I felt much better. I began taking stock of my life from that point onward. Paul had been my "External Guru" because he was largely responsible for helping me see my own sorry situation.

I began to meditate. I stopped drinking and smoking. I tried to give my peers more room to do their own things.

Meanwhile, I became friends with two other guys in my area. One of them was Al Schwab, a tall, black-haired, programmer of German descent who had recently joined the publication department. Al was another lesson in humility for me: programmers were not supposed to know much about writing, but he knew more about English grammar and had a larger vocabulary than I could ever hope to command. Al had recently attended a class on psychic phenomena at Ulster Community College. While there, he met a person who was in communication, through a process called automatic writing, with a personality similar to the disincarnate Seth personality of the Jane Roberts books. This experience heightened his interest in psychic phenomena way beyond simple intellectual curiosity. His attitude was highly contagious, and I found myself dragging out the old books and buying new ones.

My other friend had been a member of the publication group for quite a long time now, but I had not gotten to know him too well until recently. R.M., as he shall be called, was a quiet, bearded gentleman who kept pretty much to himself. He was quite deep into meditation, having practiced it for some months already. R. coupled a literary mind with a quick sense of humor. He cast the I Ching, and he played an excellent hand of bridge. He was to play an important part in validating my Kundalini experience a few short months from now.

There were a number of other people who became involved in our daily psychic "klatches," but their involvement would not be a major factor in the powerful psychic triangle that would soon be formed by Al, R.M., and myself.

To summarize: It was almost as though I had been set up for the Kundalini event to happen. The seed had been planted years ago, and the soil had since been carefully nurtured. Years of success had carved very definite patterns of ignorance deep within me. My reality was a postcard reality, peopled by cardboard figures to be manipulated and thrown away when no longer useful. I was living in a dream world of preconceived notions and predictable outcomes—sleepwalking even while awake.

And then came the turbulence that made me grab hold of my hanging strap. Frustration after frustration whipped me, effort after effort failed: the depths of despair were upon me. The suffering that I was going through was like a rock taking me to the bottom of the sea.

But suffering is sometimes required before man can get a glimpse of himself. And my meditation and newfound friends turned out to be the "spark of purity" within my suffering that grew into a meaningful spirituality: a new way of enjoying the old world—which is always and forever new when one stops to think about it.

PRELIMINARY EXPERIENCES

July, 1974, to February, 1975, was a golden period of strange, new experiences and expectations. I was not to have the classical Kundalini awakening until February, 1975; nevertheless, the period preceding the event was almost as exciting as the times to follow.

During these months Al, R.M., and I got to know one another better. We shared the information we gleaned from our books, discussing some of the concepts excitedly during coffee breaks and other fleeting moments we could spare from our work.

Each of us began to notice that we could sometimes predict what the others would say, and how they would say it. At times this effect was uncanny. It was as though we were in each other's minds. This helped to draw us together into a very tight brotherhood.

I began meditating in July, 1974, and began to feel my first relief from chronic anxiety around late October or early November.

In the course of my reading, I came upon an advertisement for biofeedback machines. After seeing this advertisement, which did a good job of provoking my interest, I began to read some of the commercial books on the subject, and I eventually purchased a machine similar to the one I had seen in the advertisement.

During this period I began recording my dreams again — a practice that I had discontinued about 12 years prior. This proved to be a wise move, as this practice later turned out to be one of the major factors in helping me to analyze what had happened to me, especially from a physiological standpoint, over the Kundalini months. As an additional benefit, the dreams reflected my desire for attainment and helped to condition me to accept the Kundalini experience.

It is during this period that my "feelies" and other psychic events begin to build up in intensity and frequency — a direct result of the growing Kundalini fires within.

This chapter discusses, roughly in chronological order, some of the important elements leading to the Kundalini awakening. There is some overlap among the items; and a few, such as biofeedback machine usage, meditation, and attainment dreams, span all of the time period, continuing even today.

Experimenting with Meditation

In July, 1974, Transcendental Meditation (TM) was already very popular, although the flood of books on the subject had not yet begun. I had not attended any of the TM classes, so in July, shortly after my encounter with Paul, I began to practice my own version, using a self-bestowed mantra.

Actually, at this time meditation was almost a matter of survival for me. As previously mentioned, my work was getting the better of me, to say the least. Stress was now taking a serious toll on my health and well-being. To continue in the path I was on would lead me into sure destruction. So out of desperation, and also because my interest in meditation had been heightened by R.M., I began meditating.

After about three or four months, I noticed that some changes in attitude had crept up on me. I began to notice people. I began to question the way I had been treating them. I wasn't yelling nearly as much, and my medicine bag was not seeing quite as much use as it had in previous months.

It felt good; it felt right. But there was another change that did not completely please me: I began to lose the self-confidence that had propelled me through problems so effortlessly before. And when dealing with individuals, I began to feel an anxiety I had not noticed before. My decisions began to lose their smoothness, to become halting. I was concerned over what others might think about how various problems should be solved. I became concerned that the meditation was not working right for me after all. Yet, in those periods in which I was not involved in transactions with other individuals, I felt relaxed, happy, and at peace with myself. I couldn't understand the disparity between these two apparently contradictory states.

But then I began to figure out what was happening to me. Over the years I had accumulated a wall of chronic anxiety around me. And the wall, which was always up, was now being melted away by my meditation. This left me exposed in my dealings with other individuals. And so, as I dealt on a one-on-one basis, I generated local anxiety that was intense during the transaction, but which disappeared when the transaction was over. And since I was now able to see both the anxiety and non-anxiety states, the anxiety seemed more severe when it came.

I decided to continue meditation, as the alternative was to return to my former state of palpitations, heartburn, and non-seeingness. And I soon passed the stage in which I felt uncomfortable with my peers.

And now it was really great! I began to look forward to having other living beings sit and chat with me. I watched the expression in their eyes, I laughed when they did, I listened to the way they said things, I felt compassion for their problems. I realized for the first time since I was a child that there are other living beings in the world besides myself. I was waking from my stupor and becoming aware.

My meditation sessions, themselves, were quite pleasant. I'll never forget the first time I sat down for 30 minutes to repeat my mantra in earnest. When I had finished, the world had lost its drab sameness. The colors were all bolder, more spectacular than I had seen them in years. And my sense of smell was heightened too. I could now smell the odor of the downstairs rug and the other basement smells. As I approached the stairs to go up into the living room, I could smell the foods cooking upstairs. Everything had its own distinctive odor. I walked through the living room and dining room into the kitchen. All of the shiny pots and pans and other metal utensils had brilliant highlights from the overhead lights. Each object seemed to stand out in sharp relief from its background. My heightened senses had temporarily, at least, put me into a new, more "sense-able" world. I even enjoyed the smell of the bag of garbage under the sink.

And of course, best of all, my meditation was stoking the smouldering fires of the yet to come Kundalini volcano.

The Biofeedback Machine

There it sat in front of me: a handsome wood casing surrounding a shiny, black panel with control knobs and switches all over it. Just in time for my Christmas vacation. I had just removed my biofeedback machine from the shipping case and placed it on the table in front of me. With this machine's help I was going to tune into myself and become a new man.

It took me quite a while to read the instruction booklet,

but at last I was ready to strap on the machine and try it out. I had decided that everything was going to be done scientifically, so before I hooked it up I opened a biofeedback log to carefully record my sessions on the machine.

During the first sessions, which usually ran about 30 minutes, I charted the previously unexplored territory of my head (no comedy intended). I found, not to my surprise (the literature had primed me), that alpha was strongest at the rear of my head, the visual "occipital" area, and was weakest at the center of my forehead—the third eye area.

I noted that I could make the occipital alpha come on just by closing my eyes and erasing all of the mental images. Whenever I visualized an object in my mind's eye, alpha would disappear, to be replaced by low-amplitude beta waves. This would happen even though my eyes were closed. At first I had a bit of trouble generating large amounts of alpha. I didn't realize how noisy my mind really was, even after five months of meditation, until I was able to see this noise in the visual and auditory feedback provided by the unit.

Initially, I tried all sorts of mental gymnastics to boost the amplitude of my alpha waves and to make them come and go at will. Some of these exercises did seem to work to a degree. For example, I would sometimes focus my concentration at the center of my head, or pretend that I was inside, swimming, my hands pushing against the surrounding water, thereby generating copious amounts of alpha.

I found that when I practiced these forceful techniques for any length of time, I would be left with a feeling of residual bliss after unhooking the machine. It was as though I was exercising new "muscles." This sensation returned from time to time, even when I was not hooked up to the machine.

After some experimenting, I realized that I could generate the most alpha when I could let go and allow my inner volition run the show. (However, the procedure of letting go came gradually. I did not completely give up the forceful techniques until some months after the Kundalini awakening.) Each time I returned to the machine I noticed that I was generating larger amounts of alpha. I had somehow learned how to do this over the time intervening between sessions.

I began to notice other strange effects. For example, after I had logged a total of about 20 hours on the machine I noticed that heat would sometimes build up directly under the electrodes on my head. This heat was usually coincident with periods of high alpha and theta wave generation. I also noticed an increase in the amount of euphoria during and after the sessions. I didn't know it at the time, but these experiences were reflections of similar, but more massive, Kundalini effects yet to come.

In mid-January, one night before falling asleep, I felt a low-pitched humming, a current, within my head. But it departed quickly, leaving behind the euphoria to which I had become accustomed. By late January, after logging 50 hours on the machine, I was recording readings considerably higher than when I first started with the biofeedback machine in late December. My training on the machine was carrying me rapidly toward my meeting with Kundalini.

Attainment Dreams

In November, 1974, I began to experience "attainment dreams." These dreams reflected my desire for enlightenment, but perhaps more important than this, they also reflected internal changes that were being caused by meditation, biofeedback training, and the consequent approach of the Kundalini event. While some of these dreams were quite uplifting, others portrayed the ego death that comes with enlightenment. As such, not all of the dreams were pleasant.

I've gathered four pre-Kundalini attainment dreams here, with some supplementary interpretation. These should be sufficient to familiarize you with the kinds of dreams you might experience on your own trip. Of course, your own dream symbols will differ from mine.

In all of the dreams presented in this section, bracketed items are clarifications or explanations made while writing the dream, or at some later date.

The first dream hints of some of the internal changes taking place within and reflects my climb toward higher spirituality.

"The Mole Men Dig a Tunnel"   *November 30, 1974*

There were many people gathered, perhaps thousands. They began to disperse in two opposite directions. Some other people and I began to walk toward

the point at which the people began the dispersion.
Someone mentioned that a very large bomb was in the
harbor water near where the people began to disperse.
Soon a small group of us had reached this point. We
were in a tunnel under a harbor and I watched as some
massive earth-moving equipment gouged out our tunnel.

We came across two mole-like tunnel diggers. They
seemed to examine the earth and then one of them
mumbled "5000 feet." This seemed to be directions for
our small group. And at this point I realized that we
were under the harbor water and needed to climb.

We began to climb up many sets of steps which at
first were large, like the marble steps in a railroad
station, but which then graduated into much narrower
steps as we got higher. We began finding rooms as we
ascended. And soon it began to get difficult to find the
continuation of the steps upward. But a female friend
of Al Schwab's met us in one of the upper rooms and
agreed to show us the way further upward.

Our group had spread out by now. I was leading,
some others were following, and Al was bringing up
the rear. [As the dream fades away, the feeling is of
success.]

The Interpretation: The dream itself tells of a physiological
change going on in my brain. (This is evidently early Kundalini activity.) It points out that there is a definable source
of excess current, a point of disruption, somewhere at the
base of the two cerebral hemispheres.

The two opposite directions represent a flow of current
into the two hemispheres of the brain. Interpreted from the
spiritual viewpoint, it represents a choice between spirituality
and materiality.

The bomb and the dispersion represent the disruption that
precedes change. Perhaps this is the origin of the Kundalini
explosion that will cause my "cup to overflow" in about two
months.

The earth moving equipment and the tunnel represent the
effect of the excess currents. A major synaptic path is being
stimulated through excessive meditation.

The moles represent instruction from the unconscious —
the biological consciousness.

The climb represents the path of the current upward and outward into the brain. It is as though new groups of brain cells are being stimulated, or "cooked," as the currents rise through them and activate them. Perhaps this is similar to the "opening of the lotus" told of by Hindu Kundalini followers. The climb becomes more difficult as the currents spread because of the "restrictive capillary" action of the brain cells distant from the source of the current.

The upper rooms are the various internal structures and configurations within the brain hemispheres as the outer walls are approached. In a spiritual interpretation, these rooms represent the various discoveries, powers, and psychic events that occur with Kundalini and higher spirituality. If the initiate lingers to examine their beauty, they will become barriers to further development (because the currents will die here).

Al Schwab is the bringer of knowledge, the desire to know, while Al's friend is the anima. She is intuition, right-brain knowledge leading us on.

The second attainment dream was recorded on the same morning as the first. Note the parallelism between the two. In this dream, ego death becomes a factor.

"The Man Upstairs Begins to Fire"

I am in a high building on a street on which there are many people in high buildings on both sides. I notice a disturbance in a building on the other side of the street. Someone seems to have rammed something into the window, or see-through wall, from the inside. Many other people notice this also.

It happens again. And now everybody is watching.

Now I am down on the street looking up at the disturbance. It seems to be a single person with a machine gun. I think there has already been some shooting.

He is going to fire into the crowd, thus killing some of the gathered people. I hope that someone gets him before he fires toward me. But there is someone near me with a handgun. He is standing right next to me, challenging the man upstairs. I try to move away from him so that when the man upstairs begins to fire I won't get hit. I manage to move away and get close to the building wall directly under the man with the machine gun. He talks

*for a few seconds and then he fires straight down into
me. I think I have died, as he is quite accurate, however I
am not sure.*

The interpretation: This dream parallels the first dream.
Again, it tells of physiological change going on in my brain.

The buildings on the two sides of the street are the left and
right hemispheres; the logical and intuitive functions; materiality and spirituality. I begin on the logical side and then
move down into the valley of neither, which is identical to the
point of dispersal in the first dream.

The disturbance is the disruption that precedes change. It
appears to be a disruption in the right hemisphere.

The man upstairs represents the coming of the Kundalini,
the approach of ego death. He is responsible for the disruption in the right hemisphere. He is the me who meditates and
forces change through prolonged yogic activities. He is
Shiva the destroyer, of Hindu mythology—the precursor to
Kundalini.

The man next to me is the ego: ignorance to be eliminated.
The accuracy of the machine gunner is the precision of the
absolute. If he wants me, I've had it.

In the third attainment dream, I am told of a crossing
over from ignorance into enlightenment, materialism into
spirituality.

"The Bridge Toll"   *December 1, 1974*

*I have just paid a toll and am now looking for a bridge.
The voice of the toll collector is with me in the car I am
driving, showing me the way to the bridge. I see the
bridge in the distance and say to myself that it is five
miles away. But all of a sudden I arrive at the bridge, and
the toll taker admonishes me for insisting that it was five
miles away when he knew it was only two. I begin to
cross the bridge, which becomes even more steep as I
cross it. But I have the feeling that I will make it across.*

The interpretation: This dream predicts the Kundalini
event, which will happen sooner than I think—exactly two
months (two miles) from this date.

The toll represents some sort of atonement that was made

within me. Perhaps it was some sort of agreement between the animus and anima components.

The toll collector is the guardian of the bridge; the higher being within; the giver of grace.

The bridge is the path for crossing over into a new life. It is the Kundalini event. It may also represent the corpus callosum, a mass of white, transverse fibers that connects the two cerebral hemispheres.*

In the last attainment dream the theme is, again, crossing over. Note the parallelism with dream three, recorded on the same date.

"Crossover Into the Crown Heights Development"

I am driving my car on a rural road. I come over a small rise into a complex of other back roads that form an "H" lying on its side before me. I cross over and begin to ascend a hill. This seems to be the back way into the Crown Heights development on the way to IBM. As I begin to drive up the hill, it seems to change into a ladder that rises in sections as I climb up. An older lady with black hair helps me to reach the top.

The interpretation: Again, the dream predicts the Kundalini event — the crossing over. The Crown Heights development is a location that symbolizes a development within my crown leading to higher spirituality.

The hill and ladder together are the same as the rising bridge in the third dream. The older lady is the anima; the toll collector; the guardian; the helper; the higher being...

It is likely that attainment dreams will always precede the Kundalini event. They reflect the unusual activity in the brain and translate naturally into spiritual attainment. They tell of what is to come and prepare the aspirant for the event itself.

For the time being, we will leave this aspect of the Kundalini awakening behind. However, there is one more pre-Kundalini attainment dream, the most important one, yet to

---

* Mystics speak of a "mystic marriage" that takes place at the time of enlightenment; Hindus speak of the female, *Shakti*, meeting and merging with the male, *Shiva*, to consummate a mystic union in the brain. Perhaps the Kundalini event establishes an expanded communication arrangement between right-brain and left-brain through the corpus callosum or some other path established at the time of enlightenment.

be discussed. This dream immediately precedes and foretells of the Kundalini awakening. It will be presented in the chapter dealing with the awakening.

Some Stronger Early Warnings

Extensive use of the biofeedback machine and meditation sessions were beginning to make themselves felt in unusual physical manifestations. By late December, 1974, I was beginning to notice a general euphoria that would wax and wane during the day. At times this had the tendency to express itself as a smile or a feeling of giddiness. I couldn't resist punning and finishing other people's sentences with witticisms.

While my meditation practice was pleasant, and had changed my general attitudes toward life in the preceding months, it was the cumulative effect of the training exercises on the biofeedback machine that was mainly responsible for the intense physical effects I now began to experience.* Of course, the biofeedback machine did not provide the spiritual values that meditation did, but it certainly held my mind focused in an alpha/theta state more efficiently than did meditation.

Because these unusual manifestations had now broken into my waking world, I opened an "Experience Diary" to reflect these occurrences. As it later turned out, most of the more spectacular experiences took place in quiet periods, rather than during actual meditation or biofeedback sessions. Apparently, I could let go better when I was not trying than when I was.

I made the first entry in my experience diary on December 28, 1974. It was after I had spent a prolonged session measuring temporal alpha on my biofeedback machine:

> *While I was lying in bed preparing to sleep, a strong force located in my head seemed to pull me upward and to the right. Shortly after that, everything became completely silent. It was as though some ominous dampening force or presence draped itself over the entire house. Everything just seemed to stop—the sounds of the house, the dogs, the cats, my wife's breath, my body functions. Even the silence itself was somehow silent.*

* I estimate that one hour on the biofeedback machine is equivalent to at least four hours of meditation.

I began mentally chanting "I am peace, I am love, I am compassion," hoping to dispel the silence, as it was becoming frightening. Soon it began to lift, and then it went away altogether.

This silent period was the first that I had experienced; however, more were to come in the next few years. The silence appeared to be caused by the brain resting after prolonged electrical activity stimulated by using the biofeedback machine. Evidently the biofeedback training was powering the Kundalini and causing these strange sensations.

On the morning of December 29, I had a dream that told of heavy electrical activity within my brain.

"Electricity Over the Gulley'

I am looking out a window at the railroad tracks behind my childhood home in Souderton, Pennsylvania. The entire gulley through which the tracks run is filled with water. I am frightened as the water begins to rise even higher and the winds and storm come up. A bolt of electricity, extremely strong, moves from right to left, going south from Souderton, over the gulley. It is so strong that I know all the electricity in the area must be out because of it. Shortly thereafter, the water rises higher and higher. It is returning from the South toward us like a flash flood. I awaken before it rips us away.

The dream tells of an electrically sensitive path that is being carved by heavy currents from the rear-center of my head toward my forehead. This situation will erupt in the February Kundalini explosion.

On January 2, 1975, I welcomed another manifestation of the event to come. I was driving home from work, generating eyes-open alpha, when all of a sudden I went into a state of extreme ecstasy that was centered in the middle of my head. It felt as though someone was pleasantly stroking a small organ inside my brain. That is, it felt like a deep, localized itch that was somehow being satisfied. It was almost like an orgasm, but confined to the head instead of the genitals. I was able to stay in this state for about 10 minutes.

Apparently, the itch outlined a path that had been flooded

with excess current over the past few days, and that had
become slightly inflamed and sensitive.

The internal fires were definitely being stoked.

The "Feelie": A Psychic Gift From Kundalini

One morning while driving to Pennsylvania with my wife
and kids I experienced a new, more profound, vision than I
was accustomed to. It was not a simple vision watched as one
would watch a TV picture: it was a vision in which I seemed to
be participating, as well as watching. It began, more or less, as
a subtle sensation of something happening, and then seemed
to bloom into an event I could see, touch, smell, taste, and
hear — a total experience nearly as real and vivid as one in the
primary reality, itself. The feeling of reality associated with
this experience led to the name, "feelie."

> *Sue had taken her turn to drive and I had begun to
> meditate. Between 9:30 and 10:30 I had three very vivid,
> rapid visions that were later reinforced by actual ex-
> perience.*
>
> *First, I saw a store with a parking lot in which the cars
> were parked double. About 30 seconds later I saw a
> black car on a side street on my right. Apparently it
> was waiting to pull into the lane of traffic moving in our
> direction. The black-haired man driving the car was
> pointing with his forefinger, like a gun, in the direction
> he was going, as though he were requesting to pull out
> in front of me.*
>
> *In a third vision, I saw a black car with shiny bumpers
> pull out in front of me, crossing the road from right to
> left.*
>
> *In the afternoon, on our way back from Pennsylvania,
> again Sue was driving. Somewhere near Quakertown,
> where I had previously had the visions on the way into
> Pennsylvania, we nearly hit the front end of a black car
> with a shiny bumper. The car was emerging from a side
> street into our lane of traffic. It lurched forward and
> then stopped as we swerved around it. I didn't yet
> think of my visions of the morning—perhaps I was
> too busy recovering from the shock of almost being*

*hit in the side. However, about one minute later I saw
a parking lot and store just like the one in my vision.
It was then, upon seeing the store, that I realized that our
near accident and my seeing the store were of the same
material as my visions on the way to Pennsylvania.*

As you can see, this feelie was precognitive: it told me of an
event to come. Since having this feelie, I've had others that
seem to be clairvoyant, telepathic, or interpretive of the internal body functions or some other aspect of my existence that I
am not normally aware of.

Whenever a feelie occurs, two here and nows, two realities,
seem to be involved—the reality in which the feelie is experienced and the reality in which the feelie content actually
takes place. While I cannot tell for certain exactly what
causes feelies, I have noticed that strong, electrical or emotional effects occur close to the time at which the content of
the feelie actually takes place (**not** at the time at which the
feelie is experienced). At such a time I usually experience
a thrill through the head and body, or an emotional jolt,
a warm emotional experience, or a burning sensation in the
crown of the head or around the ears.

In the case of the feelie just covered, the sudden shock I
experienced when the black car almost hit us may have
served to distort time and space in some fashion.

With the increase in Kundalini currents, feelies began
to creep, almost unnoticed, into my subliminal, waking
thoughts. I would find myself speaking with my friends about
subjects that I would then go on to read about some hours
or minutes later. Or I would find myself previewing my
friends' thoughts shortly before they voiced them. Very specific concepts and topics would thus "arrive before they
came," so to speak.

As I began to incorporate this feelie mode of thinking
into my daily routine, my thoughts seemed to take on more
form and substance. They had a palpable presence within.
The difference between feelie thinking and the more normal
state was similar to the difference between swimming and
walking in the open air: that is, when you are in the water
you are more conscious of your environment than when you
are in the open air. I found I could almost hold my thoughts
in my hands.

And then, on January 15, I experienced a powerful feelie that I would later discover to be directly related to my February 2 Kundalini event. It came while I was in deep meditation during my noon hour at work.

> *While meditating in my office, I had a number of animated visions in rapid succession. First, I was apparently standing outside of my office, where I became aware of R.M. He was bobbing and hopping and spinning around me, humming in a mock-businesslike manner, and bumping me on all sides while moving around my circumference like a ball bouncing off a pinball machine bumper. He was playfully working at restraining me.*
>
> *After this vision, there were others in which people were throwing things not to me, but at me. It was as if they were trying to hit some inner aspect of me, rather than the external me.*

Immediately after the visions disappeared, I stopped meditating to reflect on what had made me feel like a pinball bumper. It was this: when the steel ball hits the bumper, it is propelled away, moving faster than before it hit the bumper. There was a similar feeling in my vision. It was as though the physical, **external** I was standing still, while some **internal** counterpart flowed and ebbed within the general confines of the external me. It overlapped and spilled out from time to time, whereupon it flowed away from my external body. R.M. was interacting with this flowing, inner me by bouncing around and pushing the internal me back into the physical body whenever and wherever my two bodies were not in phase.

R.M.

The dual me, with R.M. bouncing and spinning around.

R.M. seemed to be monitoring or supervising the activity of some inner me. As you will see in the next chapter, he plays an important role in validating my Kundalini awakening. This particular feelie is a forward reflection of what will happen to R. and me at that time.

THE KUNDALINI AWAKENING

By the end of January, I had logged on 54 hours of bio-feedback time. This was pretty heavy use, since I had owned the machine for only one month. In fact, thinking back, I was probably pushing my luck to spend so much time on the machine. And, of course, the intense physiological experiences I underwent over the last half of January reflected my very heavy use of the machine.

Strangely enough, unlike preceding months, there was only one night in this month on which I remembered a dream. On January 26, I had an attainment dream that was almost classic in its symbolic offering of Grace, an event that is said to be a prerequisite to the Kundalini awakening. I include it here.

"The Advance Messenger"

I see hundreds of pinpoints of light in the sky. They are way up, and do not appear to be moving together. Suddenly, I realize that they are flying saucers. I call attention to them so that others can see. Soon they begin to get lower, thus bigger. We can all see now that they are, indeed, flying saucers. They all appear to be of the same design. That is, they all have the same insignia. [I can't remember what the exact shape of the insignia was, but it was definitely a symbol for unity— the White House, or the Washington Monument, or something like that.]

Next there were very colorful, symbolic movies shown to the world on the movie screen of the sky. These movies all implored us and asked us to live in peace with one another. The movie scenes attempted to communicate by first showing us a bad, or undesirable, scene and then changing it into a good, corrected one. The last symbol was of a large, red heart, symbolizing peace and love.

Then I was in a strange house, somewhere in the country. I became aware of a small, chalky-white man with a large head. In a strangely mechanical voice, he asked me if I could accept and live in this peace that was offered/implored. I went outside into some sort of screened-in porch, answering "yes," as I went.

*And then, as emotion built within me and I realized
I was not afraid, I said yes again and parted the screen-
ing, stepping outside in the darkness to meet my friends.*

*And now I saw a white space suit with a single, large,
square panel where the eyes would be. [This suit is the
same impression I get when I view a mental afterimage
of my biofeedback machine after closing my eyes during
a session.]*

*The wearer is a female. The face portion of the suit
separates and I kiss the visitor from space, thereby
accepting peace and love. I see other people behind
her, in the distance. It is daytime where they are. They
run and laugh in the sun.*

In Kundalini lore, as in Christian belief, Grace is given
from the One above. This higher being, who resides in each
and every one of us, is symbolized by various individual,
cultural, and religious images, according to our rearing im-
prints. The higher being can be seen in dreams or during
meditation or quiet periods. In fact, such a sighting is a
major spiritual goal for people of many creeds.

To some, He will be an image of Christ, adorned in long,
white robe. Others will see the Virgin Mary. Still others
will see white light, or a being bathed in blue light, or a
man from the stars. Some will even see the innocence and
purity of God symbolized by a little girl come down from
her house on a high hill to play.

According to the spiritual texts, acceptance of the higher
being's offer—full, selfless surrender without fear—is an initiation into spirituality. It is the first major step toward knowing
and living one's Godhood. It leads man from the darkness
of ignorance into the light of day.

And now it is the evening of February 1, 1975. Today
has been pretty much like other recent Saturdays, except
that I spent almost four hours on the biofeedback machine
earlier—more than I ever spent in one day. This left me
feeling a little groggy, but very pleasant overall.

It must have been around 11:00 PM, or so. I was lying
in bed, prior to sleep, looking out into the hallway, when I
realized that the arrangement of the room and the direction
of the bed were very much like the arrangement of the
bedroom I slept in as a child.

Soon this similarity brought on a confusion of sorts. I couldn't remember where I really was. Somehow, I believed that I was in my childhood house, and not my current one. This proved to be a very strange feeling, and concerned me slightly.

Then I noticed that my thoughts of current reality were dimmed also. I tried to think of my wife and children, but they were somehow very distant. Everything in what was supposed to be my present reality was distant.

I was in a state of extreme physical and psychological perplexity. But instead of fighting it, I gave in to it and allowed myself to lie in my childhood bed. After a few minutes, the feeling went of its own accord. Little did I know that I was now within minutes of blasting my way into the new world.

Ka-boom!

It was now very early Sunday morning, February 2, about 12:45 AM.

I had just rolled onto my back and was waiting for the oncoming slumber when I began to see a faintly pulsating light in my mind's eye. I had noticed this light a few times before, during meditation. So it did not cause me any concern. In fact, I looked forward to it. But soon the light began to pulse more brightly. Something was definitely going on internally.

Shortly thereafter, an internal query was made somewhere deep within me. It was a question about whether the experience should be permitted to continue. It was not a conscious query; rather, it was buried—almost subliminal. The query was answered almost immediately, in the same nearly subliminal manner. The decision was to go ahead—intensify—rather than cut off the experience. All of this transpired without words.

Immediately the lights intensified and overpowered me. I could no longer quite understand the experience.

The intensification was accompanied by many strange, loud sounds—discordant, but somehow not unpleasant. These were not quite understandable either.

At the same time, I felt a strong current running between the center of my head and my forehead, ter-

minating just above my right eyebrow. This feeling was quite pleasant—almost sexual.

My heart rate seemed to go way up as the experience intensified. However, I don't know exactly how I knew this, because I was no longer primarily aware of my physical body.

After this period of initial confusion, the lights changed drastically. From a non-understandable pattern of random light, they snapped into an understandable, fixed, holographic pattern of large, luminous balls. These balls seemed to form a corridor that I was either traveling through or part of.

This development was a transmutation of consciousness for me. That is, it was a complete change of the environment in which my awareness normally operates. My body-sense, with which my self had associated all my life, had changed into a "luminous-ball-sense," in which the new environment of luminous spheres was my new body.

While all this was going on, a thought welled up within me. It grew rapidly from the intensity of a normal thought into the intensity of a voice. I knew the thought was my own because I had watched it grow within me.

It said, "Who is thinking now, Fred?"

The thought was extremely strong—power incarnate. It was like a voice from heaven, trying to make a point to some Fred in my life, or perhaps even to some personality component of my own.

The thought seemed to give additional impetus to my travel down the corridor, whereupon I got frightened and became reluctant to continue.

I tried to cut back on the intensity of the experience by examining where I was. That is, I wanted to be able to recall myself being on the bed.

But I realized with horror that I couldn't focus on where I was! I again tried to make it like it was before the experience started, but I couldn't do it. It was as though the cognitive energy required to know my place in the universe was being used up by the traveling venture itself, and was not available to cognition or perception of an external universe.

For a few seconds that seemed like an eternity, I was

trapped in the hell of being nowhere, lost and frightened. But then a new development restored some of my poise.

I began to flicker, or arc, between my childhood home and a model (it seemed artificial, somehow) of my current home. It seemed as though this model was being provided to help me get back.

Finally, the corridor vanished and the vibrations stopped, and I was able to realize where I was. All of this seemed to take maybe ten seconds, but this is just a guess.

After the experience had passed, I opened my eyes, turned on the light, and, after making sure that I was still in one piece (I felt good!), got up to write down as much as I could reconstruct. Sue was lying peacefully beside me, sleeping soundly as though nothing had happened. After writing as much as I could remember, I stayed up for another hour or so, too excited to go back to bed.

It is interesting to note the various transitory stages of awareness and comprehension during the experience. I passed from normal body awareness to a state of highly confused perception of internal stimuli. From this state I passed into another state of normal comprehension, only of another order of existence. It was as though my awareness had been thrown into the air, to come down where it may.

A few of the incidents in this experience were similar to classical Kundalini incidents known by Kundalini subjects of ages gone by. For example, the response to the internal query is the surrender that must precede the event. The current in the forehead is the classical opening of the third eye. And the sound that accompanied the viewing of the white spheres is the music of the spheres in the true interpretation of that mystical event.

The classical rising up the back by the Kundalini was not experienced in the February awakening; however, this rising was to occur over the next few months.

The point at which the lights snapped out into a holographic pattern was an order of magnitude change from the way one normally experiences one's life. My consciousness had literally transferred itself from this being of flesh into an energy construction. This single event completely changed my idea of what is self.

One last reflection: everything that could be called my consciousness—that is, my thoughts, my emotions, my awareness—all of these were magnified to gargantuan proportion. The magnification included my fears and my subconscious tendencies, as well. (For example, my drive for power is reflected in my feeling of the *power* of the thought that welled up within me.) Everything mental was intensified.

It was this part of the experience that was, upon later reflection, to give me personal insight into the origins of the concept of heaven and hell being within man himself. I could now see through experience that a person with deep emotional or mental problems would be destroyed in his own unconscious swill if subjected to such an experience for any length of time. While a selfless person, a loving person, would be taken to the heights of bliss.

And this must have been what Christ and other high beings felt so compelled to teach mankind—that heaven and hell, that good and bad, that God and the Devil are known within each individual. They are he.

The morning after the experience I had a dream that featured R.M. In this dream, I was telling him something or he was telling me something—I can't remember which. This dream of R.M., the first in which he appeared, was to be a cog in the validation of my experience as something other than just a super-strong hallucination. (Unfortunately, because of my excitement over the experience, I neglected to write down the dream, and thus forgot its content.)

The Validation

On Monday, February 3, I went to work, eager to talk with Al and R.M. about what had happened to me over the weekend. Al was very excited to hear of my weekend in another world; however, R.M. was not feeling well, and would not come in until Tuesday.

On Tuesday R.M. walked into my office early in the morning. "Tom, " he said, "You'll never guess what I saw last night." R. was the most reserved of our triumverate, and I detected some nervousness in his manner, as though he wanted to tell me what had happened to him, but was not sure how I'd react to what he had to say.

As he spoke, I became extremely alert and acutely aware. (The "bright" of my past was activated.) I knew that he had seen me, and told him so. (I had been waiting for someone to come tell me that he or she had been aware of my experience, so powerful had it been. After all, at the time that it happened I felt as though I had splashed myself throughout the whole universe.)

"Yes,—how'd you know?" He said. His eyes registered shock and he seemed to be completely taken aback.

I told him about my powerful Sunday morning experience and suggested that it somehow related to his Monday night experience. But I didn't tell him exactly what had happened to me, and I stopped him from telling me his story. I wanted him to write up his version for comparison to mine. He came back with the following writeup about two hours later.

February 3, Monday, 1975 about 11:10 PM.

I wasn't tired, but I went to bed anyway in the hopes of being able to get up on time for work. J. (wife) and I talked for several minutes and then stopped. Trying to prepare myself for sleep, I tossed and turned for several minutes. I wondered how much time had passed since I got to bed.

I thought then about "time." (I was lying on my right side facing away from the window.) I postulated that our entire universe might simply be taking place in a second. I immediately challenged this: that's stupid I told myself. (I rolled over now facing the window.) Why, I asked, is it stupid? Humans' time span is a second compared to the universe's. (I used the figure 8.5 or 9 billion years at first and then reduced this to a billion.) And compared to an atomic particle, humans' time span is a billion years.

I then looked up and saw first an intense, smallish light, several times the size of a star in the sky.

*Almost immediately it elongated into a large, oval shape
either in the sky or between the sky and our bedroom
window. I blinked my eyes to make it go away. It did not.
(So far I had not really examined it to see precisely what
it looked like.)*

*I turned away, but when I looked back, it was still
there. I told myself I was not seeing it. Yet, I was.
I began to say words to myself such as sky, window,
light, to make the shape go away. I did not want it to
go away because I was afraid, I wanted it to go away
because I did not think it was there.*

*More than a minute had passed by this time and be-
cause it had not gone away, I studied it. (Even now,
I was saying to myself "What the hell is that?")*

*As I said, the shape was large, by now perhaps several
hundred times the size of a star in the sky. It was oval
in shape, but much longer than wide, roughly the same
symmetry as a Victorian hall mirror. Its color was the
same as a bright star on a clear winter's night. I could
see that it was composed of round, intense balls of
light. At the center, the shape was so concentrated as
to be opaque, silver light. Surrounding the center, the
light stratified slightly, so that the ball effect was apparent.*

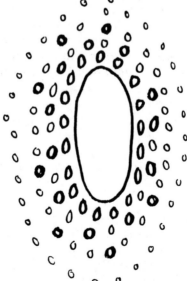

At the very edge of the shape, I could discern a slight reddish coloring around the light balls. The shape was distinct and certainly self-contained: by that, I mean it was a shape with an energy center and not simply a disorganized twinkling of light.

The shape moved a bit closer to the window. It did not so much hover or move as it did vibrate, but not a striking vibration — more like the strain of holding the shape together, a dynamic tension of sorts. (By now at least another minute had passed.) Initially, I recall, I said to myself UFO, but quickly discarded this. The name Tom Wolfe occurred to me; I stress occurred to me because I did not think about it. I couldn't understand why I continued to see it, and for a moment I got afraid, but this passed.

I turned away, turned back, it was still there, but now it seemed to be breaking apart; breaking apart is not the right way of putting it — the energy balls around the shape began to form with the intense center of the shape and then elongate, stretching so that it was no longer ovoid, but rather a swath of light that was tugging out at both ends.

The shape then moved; again, moved is not the right word. Instead of being framed in the window it was now on the right side of the window. The shape no longer held its form. It was a swath of silver light, not as intense as before, and with no discernable energy paquets. It formed an arc like the sloping shoulders of Tom Wolfe, although much larger in size than a human being.

> *At this point I said aloud, "What the hell is that?"*
> *J. looked up, but the shape was gone. She said, "I'm*
> *scared."*
> *I said, "Of what?"*
> *She answered, "I don't know."*
> *I continued to look for the shape, but it did not return.*

And so went R.M.'s sighting.

As an aside, R.M. mentioned that on Tuesday morning his wife had a dream about their pet Mynah bird, Fred. She dreamed that Fred died. But before he died, he recited everything he ever knew. This is interesting in light of the strong reference to a Fred in my experience.

It is interesting to note the parallelism in R.M.'s writeup and my own. Both tell of increases in intensity. In my writeup the increased intensity takes place just as I became aware of the white balls, and again when I became aware of the thought "Who is thinking now, Fred." R.M. also noticed two major changes of intensity, which are best described by the drawings of the images he saw: first he saw the small, intense light, then the larger light with the stratified balls, then finally the swath of light.

In my version, I **am** the event. That is, I am seeing it from the inside, with the stratified balls surrounding me. R.M. sees the event from the outside: he is a witness to it. This tends to indicate that the total event was **not** telepathic, but was instead an actual psychic event experienced by us both—R.M. from the outside, and me from the inside. It is strange, though, that my experience and his sighting are separated by 46 hours.

It is a matter of curiosity to speculate why my friend saw me in this manner. I theorize that he saw me for at least two reasons: first, he had made himself super-sensitive over the past few months by meditating heavily. This naturally made him receptive to a powerful psychic event. Secondly, and perhaps more significantly, R.M. and I were tightly bound together by our mutual interests. I suspect that people with intense mutual interests actually **become** each other to a certain extent. (You have all seen married couples who have even come to look alike over the years. This could be because their internal body mechanisms have come into entrainment, just as the grandfather clocks spoken of in Part 1. This theory is certainly supported by the commonality of experiences that will continue to haunt R.M., Al, and myself over the next year or so.

Previously we discussed two other events that should now be recalled to strengthen R.M.'s sighting as a verification of my experience. (Or, conversely. to strengthen my experience as a validation of R.M.'s sighting! After all, what is cause and what is effect?)

The first event is the Pinball feelie discussed under "The Feelie: A Psychic Gift From Kundalini." In that feelie, which happened about two weeks prior to the Kundalini awakening, R.M. was monitoring some inner aspect of me that was ebbing and flowing beyond the boundaries of my physical body. This takes on added significance in light of the role R.M. played in the February Kundalini sighting. Perhaps the January 15th feelie was powered by the February 2 event.

The second event that strengthens the causality tying together my experience and R.M.'s sighting is the dream I had of R.M. on the morning after the experience.

And so we now have an intricate web of psychic events that all seem to be part of a single, more significant event. There is:

- the January 15th feelie,
- my February 2nd Kundalini experience,
- my dream of R.M. about 6 hours after the Kundalini experience, and
- R.M.'s sighting 46 hours after the Kundalini event,

none of which seemed to relate to any of the others until after the last piece, the sighting, came about, but all of which, taken together, form a very interesting picture puzzle of universal dynamics.

AFTERMATH: THE NEXT SEVEN MONTHS

The Kundalini event was quite spectacular, but I was able to pass through it rather quickly. The aftermath of the event was even more awesome than the event itself, for now I had to get used to living in the world into which I had been thrust so violently.

My inner energies had in no way been diminished by the Kundalini event: they were still up, and would continue to be so for the next seven months. The psychic phenomena I began to experience prior to the Kundalini event would intensify over this period, and would then abate and intensify periodically during the next two years.

As mentioned before, the Kundalini experience was a massive discharge of accumulated energies—a cup running over. The raw power of this discharge had temporarily deadened some of my body functions such as sex and negative emotions. For some reason, it had left untouched, and even magnified, positive emotions such as love, compassion, and a feeling of goodwill toward others.

Apparently, it had also disrupted communications, or at least altered the normal path for communication, between the right and left hemispheres of my brain. This was made evident by the first few dreams following the Kundalini event.

Injury (Modification) to Right-Brain

Soon after the Kundalini event, my dreams notified me that all was not well with right-brain. The first dream I had after the morning of the Kundalini experience (eight days later) informed me that right-brain (represented by anima symbology) had been modified, and perhaps even hurt, by my foolish left-brain, intellectual attempts to hurry the awakening. It gives a vivid portrayal of the state I had put myself in by my hasty action. It is evident from this dream that my internal body mechanisms had been confounded.

"The Anima Atrophies"   *February 10, 1975*

I am a handsome, strong fellow, attractive to all the girls. I am lying in bed with one in a girls' dorm.

Now I am in a crowded room—perhaps a school lunch room. A girl whom I had courted and her father approach, but they don't see me. It is as though I spoiled her because she was too young for me. She seems to have gotten smaller and younger—perhaps atrophied—possibly because I didn't wait until she was ready.

Now I see a freezer—a white, counter display for cold meats with a glass window. Inside is a slab of frozen meat that represents the girl in a fully atrophied form. But then I see her walking out the side door hand in hand with her father, who is scolding her. Her father is Tom Mesick...

The scene changes. Now I find myself riding (not driving) in a car. Someone is now narrating. I come to some lowlands where there are three houses built at the end of a white brick or stone dam. It seems silly to me that people would place themselves in such jeopardy; however, I understand that one of the houses, the center one, is mine, or is related to me in some way.

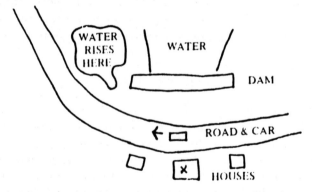

As we drive by, the narrator announces that there could be an aneurism in the dam.

Now we begin to go up a hill, away from the scene. I appear to be in a yellow Volkswagen with someone else doing the driving. I see my hands fumbling at the window curtain so that I can see out. I look back and see the water rising over the lowlands around the area.

The narrator becomes excited as the aneurism develops. He announces that the dam is going. (Something like, "Oh no, there it goes—.") However, I don't actually see the dam break or the houses go.

The interpretation: It is obvious from this dream that there have been important changes within as a result of the Kundalini awakening. In fact, the effect was so devastating that it took the dream mechanism eight days before it could gather itself enough to report on the state of affairs within.

Apparently, the dream first chastizes the logical, rational me for muddling ahead on my own. I am shown, via the image of the fully atrophied meat (my brain?) within the freezer, what could have happened to me.

The internal body mechanisms then take the anima away to recover. After this, I am once again shown the silly position in which I have built my house (put myself in).

The girl, of course, is the anima—right-brain function. Her father is the higher authority—control of internal body functions. His name, Mesick, is an obvious symbolic reference to the brain's current state of health. Something has happened to it that he still hasn't been able to figure out.

The dam and the rising waters represent the stored up energies, which are still at dangerous levels. The houses represent the beings (namely, me) who would be swept away by the force of the water (current) should the dam break.

Prior to this dream, I believed the word "aneurism" to mean "a weakness in an artery," hence the bursting of the dam and spilling over of the energies.

The yellow Volkswagen represents the internal component who takes me out of danger's way. In subsequent dreams, this component is represented by a black man dressed in yellow or orange. He will play the role of "engineer of my train," controlling the operation from within. This is not unlike the Hindu concept of the internal Guru, who leads the devotee in his trip across the ocean of *maya* (illusion).

With right-brain functions now (temporarily?) withdrawn from my total being, I soon encounter applicants desiring to take over these functions within me.

Possession Attempts

Beginning shortly after the Kundalini experience and continuing over a number of months I was plagued with a great number of dreams in which attempts were made to possess me. I believe that these attempts were from components of my own personality that were fractured from the main personality body by the powerful Kundalini experience.

The nature of these possession dreams changes over the months. Early dreams begin quite innocently with secretaries or other females applying to assist me in some way. In later dreams, a small, dark man of Spanish, Negro, or Indian descent disguises himself as a female to win my approval and gain entry. When these attempts fail, the dreams become more direct: black men begin to intimidate me.

Eventually, the dreams become more sophisticated. In one, there is a simple request to "stand on the black squares," with the implied result being that I will be zapped by electrical currents and changed in some mysterious way.

In almost all of these dreams, the intruder is characterized by blackness or darkness. Through all of the attempts, I resist. And over the seven month period the dreams slowly begin to wane: either the intruder is giving up or reintegration is preceding slowly but surely. (Later on, however, I do have dreams in which a black man resides in my house.)

I've included a few possession dreams here to give you an idea of the kinds of dreams you might expect after your Kundalini experience.

"Surrogate Anima"   *February 11, 1975*

---It is now time to fill out our forms. I notice that the form belonging to the woman on my left ranks her very high. In fact, I notice that one of the entries says

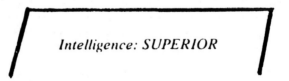

Intelligence: SUPERIOR

I have the impression that she is quite experienced. And it seems as though she has filled out the form for my benefit, as if she was applying to perform some service for me or to work with me in some way.---

The Interpretation: Someone is applying for the job of anima!
In the next dream, a black man becomes a female impersonator.

April 19, 1975

> *I am sitting in a train station waiting for some event to happen. There is a rather attractive girl sitting beside me. I have my arm around her, and we seem to like each other very much. At one point, I notice Sue (my wife) sitting across the small waiting room from me.*
>
> *Soon it is time for the girl to leave, but I have the impression that we will get together again. She is standing at a distance, saying goodby, as though she just came out of the rest room in preparation to go.*
>
> *I realize now that "she" is a man. He is short and, I believe either black or Spanish.*

The Interpretation: Hindu text says that when one needs a guru, the guru will appear, sometimes subtly, and sometimes in person. Knowing this, and by now knowing that I was undergoing a Kundalini transformation, my dream mechanism probably used this format to describe the activity going on within.

It is interesting to note that I would shortly become acquainted with the writings of Swami Muktananda, a Siddha Yogi from Ganeshpuri, India. And in 1976, I would meet him in person in South Fallsburg, New York.

I do not recall the exact features of the dark man in my dreams; however, the general size and build is similar to Muktananda's. I have always wondered whether the black man in those early dreams was Muktananda, come to moderate the Kundalini currents within me, and whether his subtle coming predated his actual coming in true feelie fashion.

It was now three months since my Kundalini experience, and in none of my dreams had I given in to the request of the black man for admission into my being. At this time the dreams began to come more to the point: I began to have dreams in which I was intimidated by black men. Apparently, I was not reabsorbing personality components as fast as the engineer desired.

"Intimidation"   *April 29, 1975*

Larry James, a black friend of mine, and some of his friends take my money in front of a movie theater. They then continue to badger me. I sit on the ground and bleat, to prove how much they've scared me. Finally they go away.

Later on Larry returns. We are playing catch in front of my childhood home. I am having trouble catching the ball, and exclaim such at one point. I throw it and it rolls way up Front Street.

The interpretation: A bit of badgering to soften me up, then—"If you play ball with me, I'll play ball with you."

In the last possession dream, the possession attempt is more symbolic, more subtle. Note also the flavor of attainment at the end of this dream.

"Temptation by the Black"   *July 6, 1975*

There were two classes of people, one which included me, being transported down a wide street that seemed to be moving us like a moving belt, or an escalator. The street looked like a broader version of the street on which my High School was located in Souderton, Pennsylvania.

Soon someone decided to reverse the belt. We were all being moved to an area up at the top of the street. There we were being compacted into a small space and asked to stand on small, black squares that had been sprayed with water to make them wet. The black tiles were interspersed with tiles of other colors, including white ones.

I suspected that if I would stand on the black square I would be electrocuted or something. I believed that the water was intended to make the squares conductive. So I didn't stand on my square until after it had dried. I hoped the instructors, or whomever they were, wouldn't discover my action.

They discovered me, but I had a trick: I could turn myself into four white tiles and by placing myself on any other four, equal-sized, white tiles on the street I could effectively become invisible. I did this twice,

*but as I recall I was found both times. (The second
time, I took a long slide down the street on my stomach
to get away.)*

*Now the scene shifts. I am riding up a darkened, foggy
street with some of my classmates. Someone is com-
plaining about the increased air pressure. Larry Palmer,
a schoolmate, states, "It's 75 pounds, twelve."*   .

*Although I don't notice the high pressure I think
that perhaps I should be minding it. That is, why should
I be any different from the others?*

*Then we come out of the fog and approach a large,
white castle, just like in Jack and the Beanstalk.*

The interpretation: All the direct, personal attempts the
intruder had made to command the right-brain functions
had failed. So now he resorted to using an impersonal approach in which he tried to get me to stand on the black
squares.

Perhaps all of these attempts are really the internal body
mechanism's way of trying to get me to help heal myself.

Descent of the White Light

My co-workers and I, all planners, were accustomed to
attending meetings on a daily basis. During one of these
meetings a few days after my Kundalini experience, Al, a
few other planners, and I were gathered together when the
room began to lighten mysteriously. A warm glow began
to move slowly downward from the ceiling.

The light seemed to be both internal and external. That
is, I could feel the warmth and radiance flowing downward
through my body, while at the same time I watched it flowing
downward through the room, softly fusing together everything it touched. It washed down from my head, into my
chest, and on down, until the entire room was illuminated
by a supernatural radiance.

I had been reading about integral yoga, the descent of
the white light,* and the downward, or return, flow of the

---

*Re:"Sri Aurobindo, or the Adventure of Consciousness," by Satprem, Harper
and Row.

Kundalini current, and was now astounded to witness this descent in my own life. Here is a February 9, 1975, account from my experience diary:

> *In the past week, I've noticed that meetings have been bathed in a mysterious glow. All of the people and objects in these meetings seem to be joined, unified somehow, by a soft, white light that seems to blend all edges and tie together everything into a single entity, or event. Everyone seems to be strung together, acting toward a common goal. If someone makes a hostile statement, it seems drained of power and dissipates into nothingness. Everything seems to feel right, and people all seem more "family" than they ever have before.*

The whiteness seemed to pervade the meetings at work for about one more week, tying together all of the participants into some sort of single unit.

At first I thought that the white light was a phenomenon that I alone was experiencing. On February 12th, however, I learned differently. Al Schwab came to our house to visit after dinner. While he, my wife, and I were talking, he mentioned that everything at work over the last week or so seemed to be bathed in a white glow. I was quite surprised to hear him say this, as I had assumed the experience to be my own, and not perceptible to others. Al's experience of the white light was evidence that the Satsang effect was quite powerful at the time of the high Kundalini fires.

By February 15th, the downward flow of the Kundalini light had completed its course, and I did not see it again.

Trying Out the New Controls

The Kundalini experience had left me with another gift: I discovered that I could achieve a high degree of control over my environment by relinquishing my tight grip on my own identity, although this might sound paradoxical.

The more I could become others and allow them to become me, the more control I seemed to have over events in which I got involved. As long as I didn't get rammy, this concept seemed to work extremely well. As long as my thinking was not primarily of myself, the miracles would occur.

My experiences led me to believe that many people who do well in their professions or avocations have active Kundalinis, and are making use, perhaps unconsciously, of this principle.

For example, Rasputin's success with women was probably due to the fact that he could successfully become them and allow them to become him. And once this subtle link had been made, how could they refuse to consummate their oneness with him? Of course, the trick in doing this successfully seems to be in **not** thinking primarily of self—a difficult stunt when sex is involved. Rasputin's morals must have been completely in line with his pleasures, he must have been completely at ease in his actions, otherwise he wouldn't have succeeded in his conquests.

And so I found that when I could "undo" myself, the incidences of telepathy and event control were high.

Soon my newfound abilities cried out to be used*, and I began to involve myself in games that exercised these abilities.

Picture telepathy: Al Schwab and I invented a game in which each of us would first draw a box, two inches square. Then the sender would draw a picture of any subject of his choosing in his box, while the receiver would try to duplicate the picture. This was fun and produced a high percentage of obvious hits. In one instance, for example, Al drew a picture of an eagle, while I reproduced the same image, only upside down.

I found that my strongest hits were made when I was able to visualize an internal light tracing the image to be duplicated. But of course, the best results were obtained in the more spontaneous setting of my discussions of metaphysics with my friends. In these discussions I would know what my friends were going to say. But as soon as I tried to force the ability in an artificial setting, it would seem to slacken appreciably.

---

*According to the texts on Kundalini, the oncoming of psychic powers can be a major pitfall for the spiritual seeker. The tendency is to become infatuated with these abilities. This attachment will ensure that the seeker once again begins to think of himself and his own pleasures and goals, to the exclusion of the higher being within. Apparently, this nearly always slows one on the path to self-realization, as the idea of "self" is self-limiting.

The Confusion Game: One day at work I was feeling pleasantly groggy and blissful from heavy Kundalini activity within. This made it difficult for me to apply myself. Later on, as I was assisting Al and another worker on a planning task, I decided to playfully project my own mental apathy and grogginess to Al.

About one hour later, as Al was leaning over a sheaf of papers on the table, he dropped in mock collapse, exclaiming that he just couldn't think. His mind felt all washed out, he said.

I was tickled: my experiment had been a success. I told him what I had been trying to do. He snickered over it, called me an "Annointed Fart," and we went about our business. But we didn't forget what had happened.

The next afternoon we attended a department meeting of about 15 people. I suggested to Al that we try an experiment in the meeting, that we mentally transmit confusion throughout the room to see if it would affect the people participating in the meeting. Al agreed that this would be fun, so we decided to do it.

It was a smashing success! We listened to one non sequitur or silly statement after another. It was complete chaos! The meeting finally ended and the participants all filed ashenfaced from the room, most of them wondering what the hell had happened.

Of course, it had been very difficult for Al and me to contain ourselves during the meeting. As it became apparent that our experiment was succeeding, we were swamped with a giddiness that threatened to break up our game.

After the meeting, however, we recognized that we had a responsibility not to do things like we had just done. Although it was fun, it certainly was not productive, and it was unfair of us to impose in this manner. We didn't do it again.

Toying with the Internal/External Servomechanism: It was about one month after the Kundalini event. By this time I had become partially, but not completely, aware of the causal relationship between the internal and external consciousness, as described in Part 1. But now I was to learn more about this relationship.

I had discovered that I could influence my dreams by

concentrating, just before sleep, on what I wanted to dream about. One night, for example, I concentrated on knocking over a paper cup with a mental "finger." That night I had a dream in which I was able to move objects simply by twirling my forefinger.

On February 25, 1975, I decided to try for a sex dream. Here is the result of that effort. (Note: The name "Jean Marsh" is ficticious.)

February 25/26, 1975   From the experience diary

Just prior to sleep, with a view toward mixing experimentation and fun, I strongly fanticized Jean Marsh and myself having sexual intercourse. Then I went to sleep, hoping to dream of my fantasy...

At about 1:30 AM, I awoke feeling extremely nauseous and weak. I had just belched some material into my esophagus, and this had evidently helped to awaken me. I felt very sick and (rat that I was) awakened Sue for her support—I didn't think I could move, I was so weak. Sue got a towel for me, after which I began to shiver and shake. I was shivering heavily and suffering much pain, especially in the lower extremities. At the same time, my head broke out into a profuse sweat.

Sue returned to bed. I shook for a while longer, then the shaking stopped. But now I began to experience severe cramps in my lower abdomen and genital areas. After two or three of these intense but relatively short periods of pain, which were severe enough to make me fold my legs up into a frog position, the pain disappeared.

Over the next 15 minutes or so, I began to feel progressively better. I was thankful, of course, but I couldn't understand why I was feeling better so quickly: the initial intensity of the nausea and weakness led me to believe that I would surely be sick, maybe for days.

For the next four or five months I was to have many dreams about Jean Marsh—never having dreamed of her before—in which she replaced my standard anima symbol, an older lady with black hair.

It became obvious to me that the Kundalini event had

greatly strengthened and quickened the causal relationship between my external consciousness and my inner, biological consciousness, and that my inner mechanisms had interpreted my instructions for intercourse as something more than a simple request for sex in a dream. Somehow, my body had reacted chemically, and was modified by those instructions. (The initial illness was indicative of the sudden change I had undergone.)

And who knows what else happened? Perhaps my psyche absorbed part of Jean's psyche.* In any event, having seen the internal/external servomechanism affected so radically by my conscious volition, I am more careful today of what I think before I go to sleep.

A New Player: A Collective Consciousness

Beginning at the time of my Kundalini experience, I noticed a feeling of lightness about me, as though I had lost a great deal of weight. In addition, I noticed a lack of the negative feelings and thoughts I used to experience as a matter of course, while at the same time all my good qualities were still there, more intense than before. My burdens had been washed away and I felt clean and pure, like the spiritual person I imagined I wanted to be.

But something else was afoot. Al, R.M., and I had made a pact to loan energy to one another when required, and to support each other through the hard times in various other ways.

Al was currently experiencing a low period that he called his "desert." I offered to take on some of his low, since my own life was so high at the time. And although the causal relationship between this agreement and my subsequent feelings is questionable, the fact remains that I **did** notice a difference in the way I felt. It was almost as though I could reach over and pull the edges of his desert down around me. Then I could dip into it, sampling it in various places to know what it was like.

I was noticing another strange effect since the Kundalini

---

* The idea of incorporating part of another person's psyche is not new. For example, gurus will take on the illnesses of their devotees. This leaves them temporarily ill, with the symptoms that belonged to their devotees, until their bodies can work off the newly acquired impurities.

experience, also. Part of me seemed to have "leaked off" and was currently at large. That is, just below the threshold of consciousness I sensed part of me hanging around, loose in the surrounding atmosphere.

R.M. confirmed this one morning. As we were sitting and talking in my office, his eyes widened perceptibly as he stared at a spot on the wall over my right shoulder. I asked him what was wrong, and he answered that he was watching an undefinable, black mass hovering like a gathering storm over my right shoulder. He watched it for about a minute, and then he could no longer see it.

What had the Kundalini experience released?!

Beginning in March, all three of us became highly aware of electrical and other physiological effects that we experienced in common, as though we were all integral components of some sort of psychic net. These effects seemed to bind us together even tighter. We began to suspect that a collective consciousness had developed among us.

On March 3rd, while driving home from work, I experienced a deep exhaustion and a nervous effect about one mile from my home. As I was driving down the steep, North Road hill, I began to feel heat flashes under my coat. I pulled into my garage feeling light-headed and exhausted.

I was so exhausted that I went to bed to rest before dinner, an activity not normally in my daily routine. Sue brought me a piece of banana bread to tide me over until dinner. (I was very hungry, as though I was having a low blood sugar reaction.)

After dinner, I went to bed again and fell asleep until just before 8:00 PM. I got up and stayed up until about 11:00 o'clock, during which time I read, watched some TV, and got on the biofeedback machine for 30 minutes. The biofeedback machine literally pinged with alpha. In fact, I had been reluctant to get on the machine because I knew my alpha was so high.*

I didn't think too much more about my exhaustion and

---

* While I worked hard and diligently to bring about high alpha states and additional Kundalini stirrings, I now backed off whenever I could sense heavy Kundalini activity approaching. This was probably due to the loss of control I experienced during the Kundalini event. That is, having had the experience, I was now guarded against losing control again. I wanted another experience, yet I was afraid to a certain extent.

high alpha production until the next day at work, when I found out that Al was so tired last evening that he couldn't move. He, too, went to bed around dinner time. Later, I discovered that Jim Moser, another close friend peripherally interested in psychic phenomena, also experienced deep fatigue last evening. He intended to work in his garden after he got home from work, but found that he didn't even have enough get up and go to read his evening paper.

I also checked with R.M. Both he and his wife were extremely tired last evening. He said that he went to bed earlier than he had in years.

Five of us, zero energy. Very strange.

On May 30th, we felt an effect similar to that experienced when walking through a highly charged field of static electricity. From the experience diary:

> *"A Ghostly Hand"*
>
> *R.M. mentioned an incident that jogged my memory on something that happened to me last night. He said that something (presumably a hand) touched him on the right shoulder at about 7:30 last night. He turned around, but no one was there....*
>
> *Last night while I was letting the cat out, I thought I felt one of the kids touch me on the right shoulder (same place as R.M.'s touch). But no kids were there. Then I thought that it must have been a bug of some kind, or a spider web, but I couldn't find evidence of either of these. Then I speculated that it might have been some sort of psychic or electrical effect.*
>
> *Al, who had now joined our discussion, mentioned that the same thing happened to him a few days ago while he was mowing the lawn.*

Another interesting, but slightly frightening, effect had been in evidence for the past few weeks. From time to time during meditation, and especially when generating theta waves, I would notice the lights flicker on and off in my meditation room. In one case, they stayed off for about 1/2 second. (When I checked upstairs with my wife she said she noticed nothing in the living room. This seemed to rule out a common electrical failure in the house.)

In another related effect, the walls of my meditation room had begun to crack loudly at various locations (only while I was meditating or generating theta waves, strangely enough).

These incidents will be covered in more detail under "The Conflagration." It is necessary to point them out here, however, to clarify the following May 30th incident from the experience diary.

> ### "Al's Got the Hammer"
>
> *Last night's meditation was very interesting because — nothing happened.*
>
> *My subjective states and machine readings were the same as in recent days, but the room lights didn't flicker at any time during meditation, and the walls didn't crack.*
>
> *I forgot about the above until I got to work today. Al mentioned that last night while he was sitting in the tub, meditating, something cracked very loudly in the bathroom. He got out of the tub and looked around, but nothing had fallen or was out of place.*
>
> *Looks like Al had the hammer last night.*

From the above incident, the idea of the collective consciousness, the common force at large, again rears its head. The Kundalini experience had conceived a mutual intelligence that was growing rapidly among us.

Soon, the collective force seemed to mature and to move from the physical world into a more subtle world. That is, the number of physical manifestations like the "Ghostly Hand" began to diminish. But, as shown in the next example of collective phenomena, it had merely penetrated deeper into our beings.

> ### "R.M.'s Out of Body Experience"   *August 7, 1975*
>
> *Last night during meditation between 11:30 and 12:00 o'clock, I had two visions of R.M. In the first, his hair was white and disheveled. He appeared to be frightened. In the second, a few minutes later, his hair was more*

natural, and in it was a purple ribbon tied into a bow.
He was smiling now...

Today I found out that at the same time as I was
meditating last night, R.M. had a powerful out of body
experience. He imagined that he was in New Orleans.
Shortly after this, he was forcefully drawn there, where-
upon he sampled the "essence" of New Orleans. But
then he got scared because he couldn't get back. He
called for help from Al and myself and was immediately
protected and snapped back by some kind of "band of
force" around his middle.

Perhaps the band of force, the purple band, and the collective consciousness were one and the same. Obviously,
some sort of collective manifestation had been turned on by
the Kundalini currents among us.

The Conflagration

At the end of March I began to experience strong humming
sounds and sensations of heat in my head. By late April,
this had ignited into a full-blown conflagration that traveled
slowly but surely over my entire head, producing many unusual effects.

The first of these events occurred coincidentally with
the content-reality end of a feelie in which my son, Robin,
had "thrown the world at me" a few weeks earlier.

March 22, 1975

Earlier this morning I looked up from my chair to
see Robby throwing his big, blue balloon at me. At
once I thought of a feelie I had about two weeks ago
in which a blue world with golden continents was thrown
at me.

And now, the balloon, which was blue with gold and
white spots that looked like continents, passed over
my head to the right, just as the "world" did in the
feelie. And Robby's body was in the same position as
that of the person in the feelie.

I was, of course, excited about this, but the excite-
ment died down quickly.

Sometime later I decided to go to the Woodstock
Health Food Center to purchase a few books on meta-
physical subjects. I spent about 30 minutes in the store,

picked up a few promising books, including one written by Swami Muktananda, and went to the checkout counter.

Just as I was about to leave the store, Mr. Blum, the owner, walked in. He did a double-take when he saw me, then he greeted me and told me that he had had a vision of me earlier that morning. (He had seen me only once previously, on a day on which I had purchased books about four or five months ago.)

As we were speaking, the top of my head started to get warm and then tingle. The discussion took on a startling vitality and was somehow very important. All the people in the store, including my older son, Tommy, seemed to fade into the background as my consciousness focused on a discussion about Kundalini and Swami Muktananda.

I told Mr. Blum briefly of my Kundalini experience and mentioned that another person had seen me in a vision recently.

Mr. Blum mentioned that he was planning to hold a meditation session in honor of Muktananda. He invited me to the meeting, writing down the address for me. He told me that Kundalini is dangerous, and that Muktananda teaches Kundalini yoga.

At the time, I thought that Mr. Blum had arranged for Muktananda to be present at the meditation meeting. But this turned out to be incorrect: Muktananda was still in the Oakland, California, area, and was not to visit New York until April, 1976. Nevertheless, I was still very excited at the prospect of meeting a guru who taught Kundalini yoga, even in this proxy manner, as I now strongly suspected that I was going through a Kundalini cycle of awakening and aftermath.

It was this excitement that brought on the warm tingle and highly blissful feeling I experienced in the store. Later, I believed that I had received Muktananda's *shakti* (spiritual initiation) through the medium of Mr. Blum, who had met him previously and was a devotee of his.

Over the next week I continued to notice pleasant sensations in my head. On March 30th, I wrote:

Over the past week or so, I have felt heavy "firing" (neuron discharge) on the crown of my head and in the parietal (rear-top) area. Quite pleasant. It feels like numerous little pinpricks of heat all over my head—a burning sensation similar to that which might be felt from putting your hand under a magnifying glass in the sun, but of course not as intense.

On the evening of the same day, I was reading a passage from *"Cosmic Consciousness"* that went "I myself have realized it (cosmic consciousness) but three times as yet—" when I felt a pleasant, but heavy current in the center of my head. The current continued for about two seconds, leaving me with a warm afterglow.

This was not just a general blissful feeling: it was a specific, localized current deep within. It returned again on the 5th of April. I was resting at home on my easy chair, the radio was playing soft music, the wife and kids were not yet back from the kids' music lessons:

Over the past 30 minutes or so, I saw many visions and had many dream-like thoughts that I was able to pull into consciousness.

At 1:55 I had a combination vision/thought in which Dr. Block, my family doctor, tapped me on the chest in a certain place while examining my heart. Still in my reverie, I wondered where the place was, so that I could tap it with my finger. But then I thought that this might be dangerous, as I don't know as much about the heart as Doctor Block.

Immediately after this, I heard and felt a loud sound/ vibration in my head. The vibration rose to a medium intensity, stronger than my visions, but not strong enough to swamp me. It sounded like an electric train transformer—like the Lionel train transformer I had when I was a kid—only the sound was lower, with a more vibrant and intense pitch.

Even while the vibration was going on, I was still able to hear the music playing on the radio. I analyzed the vibration and compared it to the music. At one point, the vibration picked up and intensified a specific note that was being played.

I wondered what position my body was in and then realized that my legs were up, propped against the arms of the chair, with my feet on the footrest. (My eyes were shut, or were open but sightless, all the time the vibration was going on. But somehow I could "see" the positions of my legs. Perhaps it was some form of kinesthesia—like a combination of seeing my position and knowing my position.) I thought about changing position to let the vibrations take hold better, but then decided against it, as I didn't see that it would make any difference.

After about five seconds the vibration began to subside. This was partly of its own accord and partly because I was somewhat fearful. Then, too, I was anxious to have it stop so that I could reflect upon it without forgetting anything that happened.

This desire of mine to write down everything that happens so that I can reflect upon it is something of a curse. It means taking myself away from the actual experiencing of life so that I can think about the experiencing—a silly thing to do, but nevertheless a habit that many of us fall into. As you can see in the writeup, I actually shortened the event just so that I could think about it! (Does a Don Juan chuckle somewhere for me?)

By the end of April, a relentless heat—a conflagration—had begun to move slowly over the surface of my entire head. The physiological effects were very strong now, and a number of powerful psychic events began to take place. I began to hear loud claps of noise, like rulers slapping on wooden desks. These noises, some of them strong enough to leave a ringing in my ears, happened while I was in deep meditation or generating heavy theta.

One night in early May I awoke from sleep with a start, feeling that there was a strange presence or power in the house. I looked out into the dining room and saw a glow appear just above the top of the lamp shade on the buffet. It was as though the light bulb was on in some minimal fashion. Then the glow went away and I went back to sleep (with one eye open). This event left me with the impression that the glow was somehow related to a man in a white swimming cap, of all things.

The next day I reflected on the previous night's happening and realized that it directly related to another manifestation in my daily life. In addition to the heat I was experiencing, a pressure was building up within my head and moving from place to place. It was not painful, but my head felt like a leather thong that had been wet down and staked out in the sun to shrink. I made the following entry in my experience diary:

> *For the past two weeks I have had a tightening around the frontal area of my head, as though there was a thick band wrapped around it.*
>
> *Over the past three days, the band has moved up my forehead, expanding toward the top and back, like a sliding door closing on a Volkswagen sunroof. It is beginning to feel as though I am wearing a swimming cap. This is evidently the result of generating heavy theta in the frontal area.*

And on May 13th, more on the conflagration:

> *A consuming fire has been moving around my head for the past three weeks, covering all areas. Last night in meditation the entire crown got very hot. To date, this is the largest area to heat all at once.*
>
> *During this intense experience, the wall behind me cracked once, quite loudly.*
>
> *For a short period of time after this I noticed a strange sensation. It was a heightening of awareness, but with a twist: it was as though I was casting my perceptions outward from the center of my head, rather than being a simple receiver of this information from the external world! But even now, as I write this, I can no longer feel the experience as it was last night. It was a new concept in perception—one I cannot easily categorize. It was an "inside-out" perception— a creative act—rather than the customary perception, which is a simple receiving of information.*

I was still in the habit of occasionally using various forceful meditation and biofeedback techniques to create heavy alpha and theta effects. One of them was a method in which I tried to focus my concentration at various spots within my head. This technique seemed to pay off in the experience just noted. Following is an entry I made in my biofeedback log concerning what I was focusing on just prior to the coming of the heat in the preceding experience:

> *Just before my head got hot, it felt as though my concentration on a point inside my head found a "new place." There seemed to be a cleft just above my forehead on the inside front ridge of the crown. After I was able to focus my concentration in this new place, my crown began to heat.*

On May 14, the external presence returned:

> *Last night in meditation I again experienced the hot crown, but not the seeing outward effect.*
> *While measuring frontal theta on the biofeedback machine, and immediately after feeling love toward Christ and Muktananda, I felt something or someone "touch" me in the head. This was not the typical feeling one gets when a hair follicle jumps due to a nervous effect: it was much stronger and more immediate, as though another presence was involved. It was immediately after this that my crown began to get warm.*

Immediately prior to the May conflagration, my biofeedback sessions had grown to one or one and a half hours long. I shortened these sessions when my experiences began to intensify in early May. But it was too late: I had already overdone it. The 200 hours of biofeedback time that I had logged in by mid-May had served to produce the conflagration and intensify my experiences, of this I am sure. I was beginning to wonder where all of this post-Kundalini activity would take me.

At the same time as the conflagration, I experienced some other classical Kundalini symptoms.

New Kundalini Symptoms

At the end of March, I was fairly certain that I was passing through some sort of Kundalini cycle, but I still wasn't one hundred percent sure. In early April, I began to experience other classical Kundalini symptoms that, with the symptoms already discussed, dissolved most of the lingering doubts about what was happening to me.

On April 2nd, while driving home from work, I was startled by a forceful thrusting and thumping about in my lower back, the *Kanda* region of classical Kundalini lore. A humorous thought arose as the movement began—it felt like a squirrel thumping about to get out. It was like sitting on a living being.

Soon my stomach got very hot and I began to sweat. At one point I had a flash of insight into the meaning behind the favorite saying of Muktananda that the guru, the mantra, the deity, and I are all one and the same. This heightened my excitement and feeling of strong devotion and brought on the desire to "speak things other than words," which I then did. The buried meaning behind this "glossolalia" seemed to be that all words spring from the same meaning and that the word, itself, is a direct expression of the one living being, no matter what form (language) the word takes on.

The movement in my lower back died down at home, while I was eating.

There are some theories that the physical vibration of chanting is felt through the roof of the mouth, where it activates the pineal gland, a small, pineapple-shaped gland that is thought to be associated with telepathy and other psychic phenomena. It is thought that the vibrations from the chanting, combined with expectant, devotional attitudes, produces the "Aaa-uuu-mmmmm" humming sound one sometimes feels in his head during meditation. It is also thought that this vibratory effect of chanting can stimulate the central nervous system to the point where it takes off by itself, thumping and bumping until sometime after the stimulus is removed, when it again relaxes.

I believe this theory. I also believe that certain **external** vibrations can produce the same effect if other conditions are also right. For example, riding on a noisy lawnmower or driving a car with a certain vibratory frequency can, in my opinion, trigger a Kundalini episode, under the right conditions.

At the time of the "squirrel" event, it was my habit to chant a mantra while driving home from work in my Datsun 510, a practice which I have since discontinued for safety reasons.

I believe that the vibration rate of this car, coupled with my chanting and my expectations for something unusual to happen, triggered the "squirrel" into running up my back, and other events that were to follow.

My mental state at the time of day when these risings began to take place was also a factor. During the day I was engaged in mental work at my job. Much of the day, therefore, I was in a low-amplitude beta state associated with mental tasks. By evening, the time of day when the Kundalini events were the strongest, my brain sought relief from the tiring beta state. It was all too ready to let go and lapse into a blissful, synchronous, high-amplitude alpha or theta state. I believe it was this high-amplitude activity that triggered the central nervous system into activity, in a fashion similar to an epileptic attack. (Some authorities believe that a high frequency of brain waves is required to take one into an aroused Kundalini state: I tend to believe that it is not the high frequency that is primarily responsible, but the high amplitude.)

On April 3rd, I again experienced the effect, in the morning and the evening. However, neither "attack" was as severe as the April 2nd event.

And then, on April 4th, more activity:

> *I noticed heavy Kundalini activity while sitting on the living room chair after dinner: a very definite activity in the lower back. After lying down for a few moments to compose myself, I went downstairs to meditate...*
>
> *During meditation my lower spinal area got very hot. I felt as though I was sitting in water or on a very cold block of ice. I also heard a strong voice and saw a vision:*
>
> *Voice: "A yank stands against a deluge of motors."*
>
> *Vision: A white flag, or perhaps a very large handkerchief, that looked like a sail. It had two sailboats painted or printed on it in red.*

I was not able to figure out exactly what the voice and the vision meant. Perhaps the voice was a reference to my unconscious resistance to further massive Kundalini experiences like the February 2 experience—I don't know.

The month of May was pretty well taken up by the events noted in "The Conflagration,"with no Kundalini movement noted at the base of the spine. But in June there were two new incidents:

June 7, 1975

Last night and the night before I felt strange sensations soon after going to bed.

On the night before last, I felt as though I was divided into two beings. Part of me seemed to snap sharply to the right while the rest of me remained where it was. Then, after the initial disorientation, the two seemed to merge again. The whole effect took about one second.

Last night the effect was similar, except my upper torso and head seemed to snap up, rather than to the right. On both nights I was lying on my back.

Also, I have noticed some Kundalini activity in my lower spine the past few days—not severe, but noticeable.

June 12, 1975

Kundalini activity again—in the kidney area and upper back. I noticed a minor stiffening of all torso muscles into a locked position, as though I was being constrained in a force field. I experienced various minor shooting pains throughout the torso.

I have no idea to what this "two-being" effect might be attributed. However, the stiffening of the torso muscles is an effect experienced by many mystics who go into religious trances or otherwise excite their Kundalinis into activity. In *"Remembering: The Autobiography of a Mystic,"* Earlyne Chaney explains how her entire body freezes into a locked position when her inner currents are up. Others, such as the children associated with the 1961 religious miracles in Spain, have gone into cataleptic states during a period of high religious fervor. Apparently this locking of muscles is common.

On July 9th, I experienced a totally new effect:

> *Last night I was able to focus very intently at the center of my head. Soon I noticed a very strong fragrance within the room, like a flower or a sweet perfume. A brief period of headiness accompanied the aroma. Later, at bed time, I noticed Kundalini tightening, but there was no rising of the currents through my back.*

The fragrance, which was emanating from within, was quite real. And I would continue to notice it during meditation sessions over the next few months.

Today's physicians will tell you that smelling such a fragrance can be symptomatic of a dangerous condition such as liver disease, a brain tumor, or the onset of schizophrenia. And this is probably true.

But whether these symptoms are pathological at the time of high Kundalini activity is a matter of opinion: Hindu texts are full of descriptions of smelling the fragrance from within and tasting the nectar. These are physical symptoms that affect the spiritual seeker at a certain stage of his development. In fact, it is probable that many of the esoteric traditions that include the burning of incense arise from this event: the fragrance of the inner event is similar to that of a subtle, flower-scented incense.

On July 28th, I had a very intense meditation session:

> *At first I thought I was going to have a fully-conscious, full-blown Kundalini experience, with accompanying nirvana.*
>
> *Shortly after starting meditation I felt intense heat in the upper front sides of my head. As though affected by this condition, the dehumidifier just outside my meditation room door began to labor, and continued to do so for the next 20 minutes.*
>
> *Just as the dehumidifier began to labor, my back drew up tightly into a knot. Concurrently I began to produce super-strength alpha and theta measured as "artefacts" (signals greater than 100 microvolts on the biofeedback machine). I felt strong movements of current in the crown of my head. Then my lower back began*

*to throb, shortly after which the throbbing moved up
into my middle back, propelled by a slow wave of
energy.*

*I was able to intensify my meditation, moving deeply
into it, rapidly and strongly, almost into unconscious-
ness. At this point I removed the biofeedback machine
so as not to disturb the state.*

*My hands were clasped together and began to feel as
though they were dissolving into one another. I could
still vary the depth of meditation at will.*

*But soon I began to get quite excited, and my medita-
tion session started to go downhill. After meditation
was over, I was left with a very pleasant feeling in the
lower-back area.*

The preceding experience is another in which strong
physiological effects were concurrent with mysterious manifestations in the external world. Whether the laboring of
the dehumidifier was related to the physiological experience is a matter of speculation: I will always feel that it was.

On August 4th, I experienced two new, classical effects
called *kriya* and *chinmay*.

*Last night I had a very strong head kriya (spontaneous
movement). My head jerked up and to the left with a
rapid outrush of breath during my meditation session.
This took me by surprise.*

*Tonight, while gazing at the floor, I saw "Chinmay."
This is a state in which one sees vibrating, transparent
particles everywhere, making it appear as though the
structures of reality are beginning to evaporate. The
effect also appeared when I looked at the walls.*

The *kriyas* were to continue for about another year and a
half. They were never overly forceful, and never lasted long
when they did come. Usually, there would be one or two
quick, strong jerks, and then they would cease.

The last new Kundalini symptom is perhaps the most
important, for it literally burned an optical blind spot into
my visual system. (Actually, it wasn't a blind spot, per se:
more correctly, it was a sensitive spot.) Sometimes I would

see bright white or blue light in this location instead of a dark spot. Although I noticed the effect mostly during meditation, I sometimes noticed it when reading or looking at a white object.

The exact time of the burning of this sensitive spot was predicted in a dream in which a simple, but unrelated, precognitive event made me aware of the more personal precognitive meaning of the dream. I'll cover the dream first, then the event.

> *"Leaving with Julie"*   *July 31, 1975*
>
> *I am doing something that turns out negative, so I am going to have to leave. Julie, the secretary, is there, and she is going to leave with me. She says we can listen to what's on the radio at 88 (which in the dream is a combination of clock time and radio frequency). When I look at the clock closely, to check her accuracy, it reads between 8:06 and 8:08. Again, this number also seems to be a radio frequency.*
>
> *She asks what station it is, I say WCBS. I look at the clock again and see that it is just a little earlier than: 8:08.*

On August 7 (8/7), one week later, the simple precognitive aspect of the dream became apparent: a notice was placed on the bulletin board saying that Julie was leaving our department.

This, of course, reminded me of my July 31st dream. I went back and reexamined it and saw that it had said that Julie was going to leave on or near August 8th ("88" in the dream).

But then, with some apprehension, I realized that the dream said she was going to leave with me! (Translated: I was going to leave, or something was going to happen to me, at the same time.) I wondered where I might be going!

I also noticed that my interpretation of the clock placed the time of my departure just before 8/8 (8:08 in the dream). And on the afternoon of August 7, after reexaming my dream, I wrote this entry in my experience diary:

> *August 7, 1975: Found out today that Julie will be leaving our department. Wonder what's in store for me?*

That evening at about 6:30, as predicted (just before 8/8),
I found out what was in store:

"Shock Treatment"

*At about 6:30 PM, one half hour after finishing din-
ner, I began to get weary and sleepy. I closed my eyes
to rest, while listening to the sounds of the TV, kids,
dogs, and other activities in the background.*

*Soon I noticed Kundalini activity in the lower back.
This was not usual so soon after eating supper, especially without meditating. It then rose into the upper back
and neck area...*

*I was almost asleep when I was struck—and struck is
the right word—by a 1/2 second surge of extremely
heavy current on the top of my head in the crown area.
It was like someone had hit me with a hammer. The
blow was extremely forceful, shocking me into wakefulness.*

*I couldn't help but think that a fuse had been blown
somewhere. I wondered what part of me had been
burned away.*

And the next day at work:

*I am feeling highly nervous while sitting in my office
(10:30 AM). I also feel groggy and sleepy, as from heavy
theta. I feel movement in the mid-back. Occasionally,
I lose physical orientation for brief periods. This is accompanied by a desire to let my eye focus go "fuzzy."
And my head is warm in the parietal area. All in all,
the effect is not too unpleasant, but is a bit worrisome
in light of last night's experience.*

The shock had done something to my visual system. From
the night of August 7 on, I would now see a bright white
disc, a blue light, or a black spot in the same position each
time I read a book, looked at a white background, or closed
my eyes in meditation.

The Sun is Up: Visions of the Blue Bindu

Most exciting in July and August were my visions of the

sun and the blue *bindu* (spot)—each an auspicious event
in the world of esoteric phenomena.

On July 18 , I had a short but inspiring, dream about the
sun. In this dream, the clouds represent ignorance; the sun
is the light that will dispel the ignorance; and the clear sky
is the resultant clarity of wisdom.

"And the Sun is Up"

*I am watching the clouds. I have knowledge of what
makes clouds go away. Then it is given to me that
these clouds will go away tomorrow and the sky will be
clear because the sun embodies the principle that will
dissipate the clouds. And the sun is up.*

There is a feeling of freshness and freedom about this
dream. Like a spring morning, something about to be born.
I awakened feeling as though I was sitting on top of the world.
I knew that something important and wonderful had happened.

On August 18, a vision of an immense, firey sun broke
into my waking life. This event brought with it knowledge
of all those esoteric passages about the brightness of the
inner sun. I now understood the event to be a literal one,
and not simply symbolic.

*As I was meditating and mentally repeating my man-
tra, I became aware of a circular patch of brilliant
light about 1/2 inch across. There was an intense brightness surrounding this round, bright ball, as well. The
"sun" had dawned on me, so to speak. That is, I had
become aware of the brightness over a period of time
before I realized that it was there. Then, having seen
it clearly for about one second, I watched it disappear.*

*The sun had appeared at the same position as the new
blind spot I have been noticing since August 7. I believe
that the August 7 event, the blind spot, and the sun
are all related.*

*Subsequent thought— 12:45 PM: I happened to think
of one of Swami Muktananda's books, in which he describes the third eye and the seeing of a blue dot,
which he calls the "blue bindu." I have also been seeing*

*a blue dot, usually when reading from a white page.
The blue dot is also in the area of the blind spot.*

*I've also noticed a sensitivity to certain shades of
blue lately. Such items stand out from the surrounding
background. The high beam indicator in my wife's car,
for example, seems almost bright enough to hurt my
eyes when I look at it.*

And a few moments later:

*The blue dot again, while reading! This time very
strong. It literally projected itself out onto the white
paper. It was slightly larger than 1/8 inch across, with
a small, black speck in it, slightly off center.*

After seeing the sun, and the blue *bindu,* I began to experience periods of various intense emotions. Strange insights and
perceptions involving other people began to creep into my
awareness. People became beautiful, shining, divine beings
for me to enjoy. I watched them with love wherever they were
—sitting on the bank of a river, working out problems at their
desks, or pushing grocery carts at the shopping plaza. They
were all divine, and things that were important to them became important to me.

One day, for example, R.M. and I were talking in the parking lot after work. He was exclaiming how beautiful the sunset
was against the backdrop of the clear sky. No movie setting
could match it, he said.

As I watched him enjoying the sunset, a strange thing
happened to me. I seemed to become an awareness without
any attachments of my own. My own hangups had completely
lost their importance for a moment, and it was R.M. who
was now all that mattered. And what he was now doing—
watching the sunset—became the only thing that needed to
be done in that moment. Love welled up within me in that
very small instant in which I lost myself.

As the July and August days and nights rolled by, I realized
that I was moving toward some end. Strong emotions continued to well up at the slightest provocation, buoyed by an
enormous power beneath. I suspected that ego death was
near. And although some part of me welcomed this, another
part fought against it. I knew that the panorama of attitudes

that were now "me" would one day be gone, that all of my current attachments would perhaps soon be no more.

There were many nights in this period that I spent sobbing quietly in the darkness before sleep to think that I would be losing my self and all my attachments, perhaps including my attachments to my loved ones. Becoming big was hard for me because I knew now that I had to cease being small. And it felt unstoppable.

Reintegration

It was now September. Over the last seven months I had learned to walk in a new world, chaotic by old standards, but breathtaking and fulfilling in its promise. But now I sensed that I was in the Autumn of a remarkable Kundalini era. Over the last seven months I had progressively lost much of the spiritual lightness that had come with the initial Kundalini experience, and now I was feeling more like my old self. On one hand it seemed like I was about to undergo ego death, while on the other hand, I seemed to be returning to my former state. I couldn't figure it out.

On September 7, I began meditations in which I pictured Christ, in flowing white robe, merging with me. Two nights later, the fruits of this spiritual exercise were borne:

> *"Reintegration"*
>
> *I awoke from a "dream" in which I was either merging with my mother or with something else, while calling to my mother for support.*
>
> *The merging continued to take place even now that I was awake. It was quick, but frightful and unstoppable: a swooping together and homogenization of another entity with myself (although upon later reflection, I realize that I was not able to determine which entity was which). The feeling of fear and resistance left quickly after the merge took place. It left so quickly, in fact, that now I was not completely certain that a merge had actually taken place.*

And now I felt the same as I felt before the Kundalini experience. Following is a note I included in my experience diary on September 15, 1975:

In this one week since the merge I seem to have it all together intellectually, more so than in the prior five months. However, my negative emotions have returned. I find myself getting angry, building karma, and requiring more sleep again. Also, today I am coming down with a cold. I do not yet know how to interpret what is now happening to me.

Whatever had happened to those functions I had lost, wherever they had been banished to, they were back again. Right and left hemisphere communication had been reestablished.

And Today—

A growing disenchantment with my position in life, what I was doing, whom I was serving, and so on, took hold of me sometime in mid-1975. By the time January, 1976, had rolled around, I had accepted a position, still within the corporation, in Kingston, New York. This meant that I left behind, with many regrets, Al, R.M., and all my other Poughkeepsie brothers in the psychic world. But we were separated by only thirty miles, and we still had evenings in which we could get together, as my residence had not changed.

1976 brought both happiness and pain into my life. I met Swami Muktananda in person in South Fallsburg, New York, in early April. As he strode triumphantly into the large group that had gathered to welcome him to New York, someone played conch shells, or instruments that sounded like conch shells, to herald the Guru. As I heard these sounds, my body thrilled, for they were the closest thing I had heard to duplicating the sounds that overcame me in my Kundalini awakening the year before.

I was looking over my left shoulder to watch him when he entered. It may have been a trick of vision, or it may have been something else — in any event, he seemed to sparkle and glow. The air around him seemed to shift and shimmer in mysterious ways, playing with the edges of his garments and making him somehow difficult to see clearly. Maybe he **was** the high being they claimed him to be.

My weeks with Muktananda, in which I visited South Fallsburg a number of times, were gratifying ones in which

I became familiar with the rich yogic tradition of *Siddha Yoga.*

On the other side of the coin, I developed a frightening yogic symptom in mid-1976 that put me in a coronary care unit for three days. This experience was quite similar to the pseudo heart seizure of Franklin Jones, mentioned earlier.

On July 25, 1976, I awoke with a painful, tight feeling in my diaphragm and sides. I sat up for awhile and then went into the living room, so as not to disturb my wife. But the pain soon began to mount and I became concerned, so I called to her for assistance.

By the time Sue came into the living room, the pain had become quite severe. And then panic caught hold within me: I feared I was having a heart attack.

This must have caused excess electrical current to be generated somewhere in the brain, because my eyes rolled up into my head and my arms became very stiff, as though I was having some sort of epileptic seizure.

Although I was vividly aware of my internal environment, I was not aware of my external environment. That is, I knew I was in the living room, and I knew my wife was standing in front of me, but I couldn't see anything—I didn't have the strength to bust loose from this horrible experience.

After about one minute of this, during which time I was held in a semi-conscious state like a butterfly on a collector's pin, I came out of it. Strangely enough, as soon as the seizure was over, the pain in my diaphragm abated sharply. This left me with a feeling of relief, but also feeling quite weak, especially in the arms. I had Sue call an ambulance, in case it had been a heart attack.

The doctors kept me in the hospital for one week and at home, recuperating, for the next. They told me that the problem was evidently not serious. It was labeled "Atrial Syncopeal Tachacardia," which loosely translated means rapid, fluttering heartbeat with fainting. (It also means they weren't able to figure out what was wrong with me.)

But deep down I recognized the cause as being Kundalini- and meditation-related. And I realized why it is that so many yogis have control over their heartbeats. It's not because they have practiced making their hearts stop or beat faster. (After all, a man doesn't fool around with his heart like that.) The first few times, obviously, they came upon this effect by accident—through their intense meditation practices.

I had overindulged in my meditation practice for so long that a form of somatic stress had entered my meditation life. Immediately upon entering meditation my stomach would growl loudly, the internal currents would build, and my body would become a madhouse of internal activity.

I began to have digestive problems and had to eat lighter, more frequent, meals so that I could digest my food properly. (I found that taking digestive enzymes and curtailing my eating after 8:00 in the evening helped my condition somewhat.)

In early 1977 I cut down on the amount of formal meditation in my life. I also reduced the length and number of biofeedback sessions (I had now well over 900 hours logged on the machine), as I felt they were a major contributor to my internal problems.

After a few months, my yogic problems began to wane, and I was again able to meditate without experiencing any dificulties.

But I had learned something from all these problems: I learned that dying is no worse than living. And while my body still fights to survive, it is no longer a life or death affair. Rather, it is something to be done while other changes go on in the world of illusion, and while God remains eternal and changeless behind it all.

My psychic experiences continue at a moderate rate. But I do not now crave these experiences or whip my body into submission to them, as I used to do. I've learned that no matter what kind of experiences a man has, no matter how many spiritual visions or rapturous episodes, he will not be fulfilled or completed by those experiences. Nothing purchased through the senses will bring him final relief from wanting or from the suffering caused by wanting.

There is only one condition that is finally and absolutely satisfying: the condition of knowing and living one's natural existence. **All the rest** is ornamental glitter that falls off in the road and is eventually covered by dirt from the boots of the never-resting seeker.

One must pause at the heart of one's activities and know one's self. Life must be lived free of attachments, free of encumbrances of the senses. A man must accept what will come. He must let his Godhead live through him. He must be fully aware in all aspects of life. He must abandon all

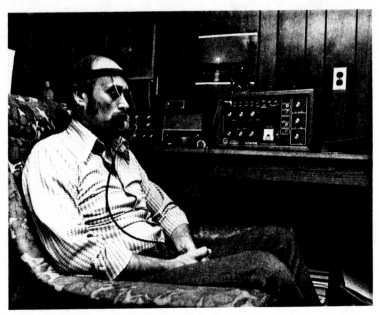
Generating alpha on the biofeedback machine.
(photo by James Bornn)

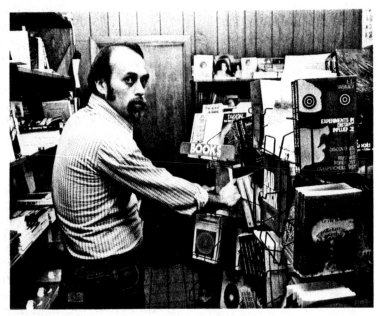
The author in the book section of his wife's health food store.
(photo by James Bornn)

SOME AFTERTHOUGHTS

I've attempted to carry you as smoothly as possible from a point just prior to my Kundalini awakening to the reintegration of left-and right-brain functions. To do this, I've been thrifty, perhaps to a fault, with the presentation of dreams and experiences that substantiate my theories and interpretations of what was happening to me during this period..

For example, I used only one dream, "The Anima Atrophies," to illustrate the changes that my brain had undergone after being subjected to the Kundalini currents. As a result of this thriftiness, some of you may doubt that I have correctly interpreted the physiological aspects of my dreams.

One of the advantages of keeping a dream notebook is that a holographic pattern of dreams and resultant interpretations begins to form after a reasonable period of time. Within this pattern, many different approaches are taken to communicate common internal problems. Individual dreams do not make full sense until they are evaluated in light of the other dreams in the pattern.

In the case of the alleged brain modification, for example, many other dreams approach the situation from slightly different angles. I would like to include but a few of them here.

In March, 1975, I began to sleepwalk and turn on lights in various places in the house. (Strangely enough, neither Sue nor I ever discovered me in the act.) One night I awoke from a dream yelling for Sue to turn on the bedlamp on her side of the bed. At this time it was very important for the left side (of my brain) to be "lit." Apparently, right and left brain functions were trying to come into a proper working relationship.

On May 20th, another approach:

"Look Ma, No Hands!"

I am in front of a mirror making my ears wiggle. I can wiggle them so that they stand out at a 90 degree angle from my head. All of a sudden my left ear stops wiggling, and I can only do my right. But soon I get both ears going again, and I am quite glad. I'm looking forward to going to work so that I can show them how well I can wiggle my ears.

The ear-wiggling dream again shows some balancing activity between right and left hemispheres. (It also seems to contain a portion of humorous chastisement toward my opinion of my newfound abilities and my desire to show them off.)

And still another approach on April 9, 1975:

"My Kingdom for a Light"

Morey Moran, a high-level manager, was going to test Al Schwab and me to see if we could fix the computer. I went down to the console room ahead of Al and Morey. I had some trouble finding the correct system, as there were quite a few systems in the console room...

I could see immediately from the neons on the front panel what the problem was. One of the bits was out in the right memory buffer section: the neon representing that bit wouldn't light.

At some point, a service routine was run. The bad bit was the only one to light. It lit in blue, rather than orange-yellow, as is customary. This indicated that my prognosis was correct.

I attempted to turn on the console desk lamp so that I could read the memory logic book to find out what pluggable unit the defective tube was in. The room was quite dim, almost dark, so that people could see their cathode ray tube displays.

But the light wouldn't go on. Al Schwab arrived and tried to find the socket for the lamp plug. The dream ends leaving me with the feeling that as soon as we can get the light on to read the logic book, we will have found the trouble.

Taken together, all of these dreams, and others like them, make the situation quite clear. They prove to be as good in diagnosis as, perhaps, many physicians would be. Not only this, but as mentioned before, the dreams themselves initiate internal activity that directs the healing process.

I have omitted other material that would have retarded the flow of the chapter on the aftermath. Some of this material could be important to the prospective Kundalini subject or to the clinician.

For example, over a period of months I had a series of dreams about oxygen, and my ability to breathe it. In this series, I progressed from a sputtering inability to breathe underwater to a fluid, rapturous, free feeling of being able to do this.

I am not sure what these dreams meant. Perhaps they illustrated my acclimation to the new feelie-type thinking; perhaps they were more specific and represented a real oxygen problem. (For example, oxygen consumption is reduced considerably during meditation. It is possible that I entered a meditative state during sleep and, because my body craved oxygen, dreamed of the requirement for air.)

In any event, they do show a gradual acclimation to this situation, whatever it might be. I produce here one of the first and one of the last of that series.

"Sputtering Underwater"   April 25, 1975

Someone is looking down into a viewing chamber or a scope hood mounted on a cathode ray tube for ease of viewing it in strong light. He begins to cough. Two people escort him quickly to the surface of the water so that he can breathe. (He was submerged while he was viewing, but this wasn't obvious until he started coughing.)

"Underwater Pleasure"   October 13, 1975

I am swimming underwater around a race track to the strains of delicate and beautiful music. When I surface, I am told I made it in 280 seconds, exactly a perfect time, and a great deal better than the 371 seconds I did the first time. If I do well in the next heats, I can't lose.

Incidentally, I am a girl swimmer in the dream. I propel myself around the pool with minute, intricate movements of the fingers and body. The feeling of solitude and peace while swimming is rapturous. There is a feeling of having conquered the environment.

There were other types of dream series or themes in this period that I should at least mention in passing:

Food Dreams: I receive food in a great number of my dreams. I believe that this represents the inflow of various energies during sleep.

Yellow: Many of my dreams feature the color yellow or orange. For example, the guru within wears saffron robes.

Natural Disasters: Many of my dreams feature earthquakes, tornados, severe electrical storms and other natural disasters. While many of these relate to internal electrical activity, some do not. These are generally indicative of losing the ego —a fear of the death experience.

Sting Dreams: During the months of high Kundalini activity, I had many dreams in which I was stung by wasps, bees, or scorpions, or bitten by snakes.

Traveling Dreams: Many times I travel to strange, exotic places, or foreign countries. In some of these dreams, my means of getting there is through a long, black vortex. In others, I travel through various natural elements, for example, great bodies of water, to arrive at my destination.

While some may believe that these dreams represent birth trauma, I believe them to be excursions into what mystics call the "astral world." They represent the travel of some aspect of my being away from the physical body and into these more subtle realms of existence.

Precognitive Dreams: I experience about one dream per month that features obvious precognitive elements. In most cases, these dreams seem to be structured in layers of precognition. That is, there is first a simple, quickly-verifiable precognitive message. Buried under this is a longer-term precognitive message. It is as though the simple, sometimes blatant, message is provided to alert me to the longer-term precognitive aspect of the dream.

I hope to be able eventually to devote an entire volume to precognitive dreams.

Classroom and Learning Dreams: During the Kundalini months, I experienced a high incidence of dreams in which I was either teaching a group of people or being taught myself, usually in a classroom environment. Some of these learning situations were quite mystical, leaving me with a waking feeling that I had learned something very important. For example, in one particularly beautiful dream I was teaching a class about a tree growing out back in my woods. There were three seasons of the tree: the first was an experiential season; in the second season the tree became edible; and in the third, it became somehow statistical. The tree was due to become edible any day.

In Part 2, I provided a Kundalini map of my own land to show the points along the way in the most interesting, most rewarding, 7-month journey of my life. While it should give you an excellent idea of some of the kinds of places to which you can travel, it is not **your** map.

Your land is your own—and your trip will be completely different from mine. And experiencing it yourself is a completely different dimension from reading about it.

So untie your rigid belief structures and skirt past the guardians of the Kundalini gates. Record your experience. Savor it. Write to me about it. And then forget it and experience life afresh.

PART 3: KUNDALINI YOU

PROLOGUE TO PART THREE

When I was young, I had a tendency to live life vicariously.
I daydreamed in school; I read comic books and science
fiction books incessantly; I fanticized myself in the positions
of my heroes.

My father, an earthy, hard-working man, noticed this trend
and carefully nudged me away from the vicarious life.

He used to say, "Wish in one hand and shit in the other:
see which gets filled the quickest."

A bit crude maybe. But from the heart, and more valuable
to me than any year of Sunday mornings...

It is not that Western man refuses to work: it is that he has
so many things available to him that he does not have time to
do them all. And so in many cases he contents himself with
reading and wishing.

For Western man, in particular, Kundalini is earned by
doing. Let the essence of the above message from a wise
father be the cornerstone of your approach to raising the
Kundalini.

INVOKING THE KUNDALINI

Most esoteric literature states that you can't force the Kundalini to awaken—that she will awaken in her own time. In a sense, this is true: until you reach a certain stage of development, the Kundalini cannot be awakened. However, there are a number of very specific things you can do to condition yourself to be more receptive, and perhaps more attractive, to the Kundalini force.

You now have everything you need to dwell in a highly active Kundalini state. What stops you from attaining it is simply your own self-imposed limitations: obstacles that you, yourself, have placed in your path.

The techniques covered in this chapter can help you to remove these obstacles if you practice them faithfully. As you practice, you will watch your limitations drop away, one by one. Strange and unusual occurrences will then become commonplace for you as you advance toward your meeting with the Kundalini.

But before you embark into your new world, you should carefully examine your reason for wanting a more active Kundalini: unless your reason is valid and your determination firm, the risk you take might be out of proportion to the reward you seek.

THE Reason for Summoning the Kundalini

There are any number of reasons why you might want to hasten the advance of the Kundalini. For example, you may want to:

- read other men's minds,
- see into the future, the past, or another place in the present,
- control other people's actions,
- become super-intelligent or incredibly quick with your mind,
- obtain wealth,
- move things with your mind, or
- visit alternative worlds.

and although you will see some of these come to pass in your life, **none** are good reasons! Each is a form of glitter with which you will be fascinated at first, but which will eventually lose its charm, leaving you back where you started — with a hole in your life: a void that cries out to be filled.

It is a curse upon man that everything he views as **extraordinary** soon-becomes **ordinary**. Familiarity breeds disenchantment. When this happens, something else must be obtained. Man again needs a new toy to keep his mind off the fact that something is missing from his life.

So man wanders from goal to goal, first achieving, then realizing that the goal wasn't so juicy after all, then seeking a new goal, then achieving it, then again suffering disenchantment, and so on, and so on, and so on. It is an eternal rush away from suffering toward a happiness and contentment that just cannot be obtained in this manner.

Let's take a closer look at the extraordinary-to-ordinary trap to see what it is that we really want.

When a person is a child, there are no goals. The child lives freely and naturally, enjoying or suffering the moment only. But the older he gets, the more he begins to live vicariously through his mind's desires. He learns how to leave the here and now to dwell continually in a wish for something better. He recognizes his basic condition as being ordinary, but his wish is for something extraordinary.

We all do it. As we slave away at work, for example, we dream of sitting on a river bank somewhere, catching the big ones. And then one day we get the vacation we dreamed about. And before we know it, as we sit on the river bank catching the big ones, we wonder what's going on at the office, or at our girl friend's house, or at any other place and time where we aren't. It seems our minds crunch on relentlessly, trying always to take us away from where we are.

It is no different with the spiritual or psychic gifts given by the Kundalini. A short time after we realize that we can see into the future, for example, the glitter falls off. We are absolutely back where we started.

Or perhaps we see a vision, more real than life, of Jesus Christ, the Mother Mary, or God, himself. And we are enraptured. We are taken to the heights and changed so that we are never again exactly the same. But then one day, after we have come down from the heights, we realize that although we have seen, nothing has changed radically, or fundamentally. We realize that we are basically the same as before. We are not filled, not satisfied. The itch again grows and we must have something else—another sign—or else we begin to suffer and doubt.

What is it that man really wants? What is it that will satisfy his desire once and for all? What will fill that gnawing void that flows throughout his being, causing him to plod ever forward toward that nebulous heaven he thinks he wants? Is there nothing that can change man's basic condition—fulfill all his desires? What is this restlessness that disguises itself as countless desires for countless objects? And why does it hide from us? Is there some malicious deity that plays with our hearts as we would play with toy soldiers, never allowing us the final victory?

The answer is simple, but to see it you need to erase your idea of self as being separate from the universe you live in.

There is no maliciousness in the scheme of things. What you really desire hides only because what looks is not real. That which thinks, that which reasons, that which builds clever descriptions of itself, is not the self. But the delusion that it is covers over who you really are and creates the gnawing hunger to know yourself.

You desire to know yourself.

And what is the role that Kundalini plays?— From a practical standpoint, man cannot know himself until all the distractions and false notions that prevent him from doing this are removed. When all the noise has been dealt with, he is then in a good position to just give up and let his Godhead shine through. Kundalini will provide massive distractions, "higher" spiritual and psychic episodes. It will expose the cyclic drama of the extraordinary-to-ordinary syndrome by showing you the folly of chasing after anything, including so-called "spiritual experiences."

It is for this reason that Western man, in particular, should chase the Kundalini—because (in addition to the very real physiological changes it brings on) it is a relatively quick means of playing out the distractions and knowing who you are. The individual Kundalini events themselves are not important: the understanding they eventually help to uncover is.

In summary, if you don't want to know who you are, or rather if you are not ready to know who you are, let Kundalini lie. If you want to remain as an illusion dwelling in an illusion, and to die having been only an actor, put down this book and all others like it. Losing the small self is a painful experience, a death. And in the end it is not really necessary because you are already eternal, whether you like it or not.

But on the other hand, if you want to know what is your heritage as a being, if you want to become **aware** in life, Kundalini is for you. If you choose the death of the small self—all those false notions and blind, egotistical attitudes—you will become the large self in life. No more desires will be necessary. You will reside in perfect comfort for the first time ever. Your restrictions and limitations will all be dissolved and God will have become you. This is what you will eventually obtain through the Kundalini.

Obstacles to the Kundalini Awakening

The Kundalini event is said to be the point of no return in the spiritual adventure. It is the "baptism by fire," the initiation into a fulfilled selfhood. Once Kundalini has come, you are well on your way to knowing yourself.

There are a number of self-imposed obstacles that delay the Kundalini or prevent it from coming altogether. While I cannot guarantee that removing these obstacles will always trigger a Kundalini awakening in one who expects it, I can say with some degree of assurance that people in whom these obstacles are **not** removed will not experience the Kundalini awakening. Or worse yet, if by some chance they do see Kundalini, it will be through the windows of Hell.

While these obstacles are not rampant in all Westerners, they do personify the stereotyped man bred and raised in an overly-materialistic society.

Insensitivity. Many Westerners are insensitive. The glamour of the gaudy world of objects has blinded us to the subtle events that take place within us. We are unable to experience our own inner beings because our attention is continually diverted to the more spectacular world of external objects. Our day-to-day existence is a loud, noisy, ceaseless panorama of distractions in which we are bombarded continually by materialistic glitter designed to attract our attention for the sake of materialism's God, Money.

And this is a vicious trap. Such a course forever requires bigger and better extravaganzas to titilate our feelings, to evoke a reaction within us. And so we become increasingly insensitive to the stimuli of the "ordinary," bored with the whole arrangement because we have run out of extraordinary things to excite us.

In truth, all the feeling you have ever expressed is a product of your own inner being. Love, for example, is contained within you in unimaginable quantities. It is boundless—waiting to bubble forth. And it doesn't need an object, another person, a target, to summon it forth. It can spring up by itself at any time, if you let it, because it is within you to express whatever you want to express.

But we have learned to attach these boundless pools of feeling within us to objects—things in the external world. We mistakenly believe that love, to use the same example, comes only with "that girl," or "that guy," or "that God." And with our attitudes toward improving our lifestyles, having more and better objects, it has become more and more difficult for us to feel and express love because we have attached it to these improved, super-beautified objects, and have become insensitive to lesser stimuli.

The obstacle is the wrong idea that feeling must be attached to external objects or to services performed for us. We need to learn to detach our feelings from objects so that we can look inward without distraction to perceive activity that is below the conscious threshold. We must dissolve our insensitivities.

Being able to feel the first stirrings of the Kundalini will, of itself, strengthen those inner currents.

Separatist Beliefs: In the Western way of thinking about things, man is separate from God and from the universe that spawned him. In making this distinction, Western man has turned himself into an object to be looked on and tossed about, as any other object. Not only does he think of others as objects, he even thinks of himself as an object.

To solve any personal problem, Western man must go to someone else for the solution: he will not take the responsibility himself. He "externalizes" all his vital attributes, and by doing so, throws away his natural abilities and his capacity to think, experience, or do for himself. He externalizes everything; he **purchases** everything.

And so, rather than approaching God through his own

being, the only place where he can realize God, he instead asks other men to give him God; rather than healing himself when he is sick, he asks the doctor or psychiatrist to "fix" him; rather than learning how to do things on his own, he asks a specialist to teach him how. Today's Westerner must even be protected from his own inadequacies by an unending stream of officious government regulations to ensure his well-being. Apparently, the individual is no longer qualified to act with common sense.

Western man has left nothing within himself! He has chucked it all out: it is "other." He has thrown away his natural divinity and become a sinner. He has banished himself from his own being, his own universe.

And now he looks to the stars on dark nights and bewails his lonely existence. He curses the God who has forgotten him, when in reality it is he who has forgotten God.

The obstacle that must be removed is the wrong idea that we are individuals apart from God and the universe.

Unreceptivity to New Experience: Our culture has stressed that objectivity and scientific proof are necessary before an event can be classified as real and included in our collectively agreed-upon reality. Western man holds rational, logical, linear thinking on a pedestal, while he confines intuition to a minor role if he permits it to function at all.

Unfortunately, absolute reality can only be known through the eyes of intuition. The completely logical, rational man can know only illusion. He will search for his smallest particle or his most distant star without ever finding it, for it does not exist in the relative universe. He is forever restricted to dealing with the changes and perturbations that ride upon the formless reality. He will never be able to deal with the changeless, eternal reality beneath the illusion.

The logical mind is "past-bound." It forms conclusions based on past events and their results. And once these ideas of what reality is about are formed, they are cast in concrete. They then act as filters that prevent man from seeing anything that does not conform to his preconceived rules of nature.

The older such a man gets, the less he can see afresh. Until one day he can see no more, and he spends the remainder of his life living like a grooved record that can play only one song.

The logical mind constructs impenetrable belief structures that act as walls to new experience. The sphere of such a man's personal universe shrinks and shrinks until no new experience is available to him and he is dead in life. Such a man must learn how to untie his belief structures to once again breathe the fresh air of new experience, for as he is, he is unable to recognize Kundalini as a possibility.

Two obstacles must be removed: first, our granite-walled belief structures must be undone. Second, our tendencies to close down the perceivable universe through our rational thought processes must be eliminated.

Unanticipatory Attitudes: Man's insensitivity and lack of receptivity to new experiences are major contributors to an attitude in which nothing is new—no more surprises are expected.

When man begins to remove the obstacles of insensitivity and unreceptivity, another obstacle—that of being unanticipatory—will automatically fall away.

The ability to dwell in an attitude of eager, joyful expectancy is one of the most important qualities a Kundalini aspirant must have. One must foster an atmosphere in which each breath of life is awaited with as much wonder and awe as the first. Each event must be welcomed as completely new; it must be examined for its unknown qualities, as a child would examine it. The unknown must not be feared, but looked forward to for its delightful uniqueness.

The eternal feeling must be one in which **something is going to happen.** And then it will.

Lack of Love and Compassion: Many of us lack love and compassion. Our continued wars and violence on the streets attest to this.

Man, in his smallness, has learned to evaluate everything in terms of its worth to him. He runs everything through a filter of "Do I want it, or don't I? Will it harm me, or benefit me? Should I accept it, or reject it?"

Acts of rejection, fights, arguments and the like, are the banners of the small being—the pocket of consciousness that has wound about itself tightly and declared its sovereignty from the mother being. Such acts show a reluctance to let things happen as they will. They show a reluctance to the natural flow of the force—love—that binds the universe into a single, coherent being.

The loving man, the compassionate man, is the "meek" of the Bible. He sees and permits the natural flow to express itself, which is an act of love, and he understands it, which is an act of compassion. He is a vehicle and a witness for the boundless love that flows through all.

Love is expressed when man surrenders to the higher being within. It flows freely when one releases his egotistical concerns. When love flows, fear is gone because there are no concerns of the small ego that it might lose something precious to it.

If one wants the Kundalini, he must learn how to surrender to love. Again, the obstacle to be removed is the wrong idea that we are individuals other than in God.

Removing the Obstacles

As mentioned, it has been wrongly taught that nothing can be done to cause the Kundalini event to happen. In a literal sense, it is true that the classical event itself cannot be planned for and turned on at will, as you would turn on a water faucet. However, much can be done to make yourself sensitive, selective, receptive, and loving, as well as to ready the physical body for the event. Proper effort can pave the way and thereby hasten the advance of the Kundalini.

It has also been stated that no two men's paths are ever the same—that a specific, personalized map to Kundalini experiences cannot be prepared for the advocate. This, too, is true in the literal sense. For example, formal meditation techniques will differ from person to person, according to individual tastes and tendencies. So too, the selection of the most fruitful yogas will depend on the individual's tendencies, as will the selection of mantras, the divinities to be worshiped, and so on.

But in all cases, **the preparations of the body and the mind are the same.** To hasten the safe advance of the Kundalini, the subject must become **sensitive** to small, internal stimuli. He must also learn to discriminate between desirable and undesirable stimuli: he must become **selective.** He must make himself more **receptive** to possibilities, he must open his mind. He must learn how to look upon the universe with the right **perspective of self,** and be filled with love and compassion.

Note that I am not teaching "Kundalini yoga, " per se. That is, I do not get into any work on *asanas* (postures), or specific breathing excercises, as does Kundalini yoga. Neither do I suggest specific methods of worship, or deities to be followed: these must reflect your own preferences.

I plan to expand on this chapter in another book specifically devoted to achieving the Kundalini awakening. For the time being, however, the details provided herein will suffice. Expect the miracle to occur! If you practice faithfully, with anticipation and determination to achieve the awakening, this is all you will need.

Sensitivity and Selectivity: You hear the knock at the back door when all is quiet in the house, but when the TV is playing loudly and the kids are running from room to room, you might miss the knock. When you become both sensitive and selective, you can hear the knock under almost any circumstance.

The first step is to learn how to eliminate distractions— to learn how to go into the stillness within you. Almost any form of meditation, practiced daily, will help you do this. And within three to six months from the day you begin to meditate, you will be able to still your noisy mind within minutes after you begin your meditation sessions.

But becoming still is not all that is required. Meditation will make you still, but will not necessarily make you selective. What you want to be able to do is still all of the unwanted distractions while retaining the ability to hear the quiet knock when it comes. You want to develop the ability to tune in to selected stimuli. And you can do this, you can groom sensitivity and selectivity together, by combining your meditation practice with other techniques.

An excellent way to improve your selectivity, as well as your sensitivity, is to **write about what you experience.** Keep records of your dreams, your interpretations, and the things that happen to you during your quiet periods and meditation sessions. This sounds like a simple thing to do, and perhaps you might at first question its fruitfulness. But try it. You will soon be amazed at how your internal perceptions have been sharpened.

I first began by writing down my dreams in 1961. I did

this for about one year while at the same time learning how to interpret my own dream symbols. Then I dropped the practice until about mid-1974.

Since dreams are probably the first place in which you will notice psychic happenings and other Kundalini-related occurrences, dream interpretation is a good starting place for establishing your writing techniques. Your first payoff should be within three to six months from the time you start keeping records. Perhaps you will begin to recognize predictive elements within your dreams, or perhaps you will tune in on a close friend or member of the family.

Some people claim that they do not dream. But this has been proven false: everyone dreams—it's just that some people don't remember their dreams. A dedicated effort to write down your dreams as soon as they occur will help you to remember more of them. And the more you write, the more you will remember, until one day you will become so proficient that you will look for methods to help you cut down on the amount of time it takes you to write them.

Keep practicing, and soon your remembered dream world will become rich in realistic adventure. Some of your fondest memories will be dream memories!

The key to understanding your dreams rests within yourself. Once you have some understanding of the subject, **no one can interpret your dreams as well as you.**

It is useful to construct a catalog of your own personal dream symbols and what they mean. For example, a boy from your childhood, Icky Squeezawart, might represent ugliness to you. Whenever you see Icky in a dream, perhaps you are being notified of some ugly situation in your life. Or perhaps your school had a football hero that made all the girls swoon. He might represent a desire to attract the opposite sex, and so on.

In constructing your catalog, simply write down what you think a particular symbol means to you. Over a period of time, you will be able to tune your catalog to make it more accurate and keep it up to date. This practice will help you to learn quite a bit about yourself—your physical and mental condition—and will lay the groundwork for interpreting the more complex Kundalini-related dreams.

After a period of familiarization with dream interpretation techniques and personal symbology, you will develop the ability to distinguish among dreams that are telepathic, pre-cognitive, indicative of illness, problem solving, wish ful-filling, communications from other beings, trips into alter-native universes, or conveyors of your "astral body" to distant places or times. The dimensions of your being will expand with the development of your new means of communicating with yourself.

I can't begin to do justice to the fine art of dream inter-pretation without completely digressing from the main sub-ject — Kundalini. I recommend that you purchase one or more good books on the subject (refer to the bibliography) and get to work: your dreams will provide the clearest and largest window through which to view the psychological and physi-ological effects of your Kundalini experiences.

The fruits of sensitivity and selectivity training are usually first noticed in dreams. But soon thereafter, Kundalini-rela-ted experiences begin to make their way into your meditation and quiet sessions, and finally into the wakeful awareness of everyday life.

Keep the pressure on: start a meditation experience diary to keep track of the various happenings and extend the sen-sitivity and selectivity enhancements into your waking life. With continued practice, you will soon find yourself be-coming remarkably sensitive and selective, partly due to meditation and partly due to the benefits provided by keeping your meditation diary.

If you are lucky enough to own or have access to a bio-feedback machine, keep a biofeedback log, too. I can't stress enough the importance of keeping your own logs and diaries to enhance your sensitivity and selectivity and speed the arrival of Kundalini.

Receptivity: In *"Seth Speaks,"* Jane Roberts explains how our own beliefs act as discriminatory mechanisms to pre-select the events we are able to see and thereby prevent us from experiencing events that don't fit into our belief structures.

Mankind, as a whole, forms a consensus, or agreed-upon, set of limitations in which reality is permitted to operate. This consensus permits us to experience certain standard aspects of reality, but prohibits all but the gifted from seeing some of the more esoteric aspects.

Individuals form their own consensus realities, too. We create our own individual belief structures that are based on our past experiences. As we get older, we begin to learn how to non-see as our belief structures get tighter and stronger. We begin to get stodgy and repetitious in the way we solve problems and perceive the world. We categorize everything that happens to us in buckets, or files, we have previously defined. Anything that cannot be easily categorized is dismissed before the reflective portions of our brains can even begin to work on it: we don't even see these new events.

Unfortunately, a large part of the problem appears to be physiological. Our brains become habitually grooved into specific problem solving routes that are activated in response to all external problems. That is, once we have learned how to solve a problem, we tend to solve all problems with the same procedures and the same circuitry. This process, a survival aid provided by nature, makes us act more like machines than like people. We lose our natural creativity, we lose our ability to examine **all** aspects of a problem, we even lose our ability to **see** all the aspects of a problem. This process, in which problem variables are gathered and averaged, takes place to help us solve problems quickly in a fast moving world. Unfortunately, it also prevents us from ever seeing the world as it is.

Being receptive means beating the automatism of the rigid belief structures and the habitual problem-solving circuits within the brain. It means lifting one's self from the situation in which these automatic mechanisms and belief structures take over and tell us what we do or do not see. It means seeing more of the ingredients that go into a specific problem.

Being receptive also means that the decision-making process is changed. As one makes himself more receptive, he moves from his former non-receptive state, in which he made snap decisions based in illusion, through an indeterminate period of confusion, in which he may be reluctant to make many decisions. Eventually he will come into a state in which he again makes decisions, but now they are based in intuition as well as logic. Further, such a receptive person is now untrammeled by worry over the results of his decisions. And as you might guess, with the weight removed from his shoulders, he is now more likely to make "right" decisions than "wrong" ones.

The receptive person throws away all preconceived notions about how things must work because of natural law. Therefore, the more receptive one is, the less judgemental one is. There are no "That cannot happen's" or "It'll never fly's" in the receptive person's vocabulary. (For as soon as one makes a judgement, he automatically shuts off the perceptive input to and the reflective processing of the problem.) A combination of eager anticipation and receptivity will ensure that the advocate sees Kundalini as soon as the other ingredients fall into place.

But how does one make himself more receptive so that he can perceive the Kundalini effects more clearly?

Meditation, worship of a deity, chanting, biofeedback training, and other yogic exercises act naturally to remove psychological and physiological obstacles to receptivity. Psychologically, they help to uncover some of the rigid belief structures so that the subject can deal with them. Physiologically, they burn away the old grooved problem-solving circuitry in the brain and allow the subject to again see things anew.

And this is why you must **practice** these things, rather than just read about them and wish that they would happen. You will change slowly, but surely, into the person you want to be only if you work at it.

A note of caution here—if you approach the task with too much enthusiasm, as did I,—if you meditate too much, for example—you will go through a prolonged period of chaos and confusion before you attain clarity. You will seem to have difficulty in making even simple decisions for a period of time because your habitual problem-solving circuitry will undergo change too rapidly. But fear not. You will eventually attain a state of clarity that you have not experienced since youth. This will make it more than worth the temporary discomfort you may experience.

Receptivity can be helped along by other practices, as well. For example, you should saturate yourself with books on yoga, natural healing, psychic phenomena, various religions, meditation, and other aspects of metaphysics. But remember that your reading should supplement your practice, not replace it.

It will also be helpful to read other types of books with looser laws of reality. For example, if you can develop a taste for science fiction, you can further open your belief structures, thereby making yourself more susceptible to the Kundalini effects.

It is very important **not** to make critical judgements on everything you read! Accept what you can. What you cannot, you must let pass in one ear and out the other without throwing the book down in disgust. You must forgive books as you forgive people, for all books have something to say, some truth to express, as do all people. And each act of unforgiveness on your part, whether it be directed toward a person or a book, will reinforce your tight, restrictive belief structures and make you smaller and more limited in your perceptions. Open up to the world around you. It is just being created now.

Self-perspective: *The ego is King! Long live the ego!*
Such is the ego's attitude toward itself.

Each of us has the idea that self is centered within the body, and that it extends outward to the edges of the body, where it stops abruptly. Having thus defined the self, each of us then goes on to attach an "importance" value to self and other objects. We first look at self and say, "This is by far most important." Then we drop down a couple of magnitudes to begin assigning the importance attribute to all other objects in the universe.

This is an act of the ego and is wrong for at least three major reasons. First, the self doesn't stop at the edges of the body. In fact, the self doesn't even **start** within the body. The self is centered throughout the entire universe and through all time. Human life "peoples" on the self like leaves grow on a tree.

Second, because the self is omnipresent and omniscient, there is no real value difference among any of the objects, any of the forms of God, in the universe. All are truly equal in God. Not just people, but animals, insects, vegetation, and even rocks, have equal divinity, equal place in the universe.

Everything that now exists also existed "in the beginning." Nothing that is created anew has any inherent reality **as** the object that it appears to be. The reality of each object belongs to the "stuff" of which it is made.

There is a story about a servant who did a good turn for

his King. As a reward, the King offered him his choice of one of two gold statues. The first was an elephant, about two inches high and weighing ten pounds; the second was an enormous snake coiled around a stick, the entire affair weighing about 80 pounds. The servant chose the ten-pound elephant. When the King asked him why he didn't choose the more valuable piece he said, "Because I don't like snakes."

Like the servant who chose the elephant, we assign values to each of the objects in our universes. We grant them their realities based on their outward appearances, but not on their common, inner self. And so we compare each piece in the universe to all the other pieces: equality is non-existent for us.

The third major reason that the ego's tendency to over-inflate its own value is wrong is that this is the origin of fear within man. A man without an ego is fearless. He has nothing to lose and, therefore, nothing to be frightened about. But the larger one's ego is, the more fear there is of loss, destruction, evil, and other worries that only the greedy, self-inflated soul can possess.

Earlier I mentioned the presence of the adverse forces, a Hindu concept that parallels, roughly, the Christian concept of the devil. The adverse forces operate on man's ego. The size of the ego and the strength (and effect) of the adverse forces is directly proportional: the larger the ego, the stronger the adverse forces, and the greater the fear generated.

There is perhaps no event on earth as completely shattering as a highly active Kundalini in a fearful man. Luckily this doesn't happen often, as the adverse forces will chase the ego-filled man away from the Kundalini event.

The prospective Kundalini subject must put himself in proper perspective with the universe. King Ego must be subdued so that surrender to the Kundalini can take place. But the task must be approached indirectly because it is the ego that is doing the approaching. And of course the ego would not think of doing itself in when push comes to shove. No, ego would play games but then stop short when the time comes to make the jump. For each man has it in his mind that he will have the best of two worlds. He would retain his small self while winning over the larger self.

So the task must be approached indirectly. To do this, you must instill in yourself the idea that there is only one being, and that it permeates all that is. **You must practice,**

**again and again, letting go of your small self to let the larger
being within take its rightful place.** As this truth begins to
grow and things slowly work into proper perspective, King
Ego will dwindle naturally. And before he suspects what is
going on, he will poof into nothingness, leaving only larger
self.

Some of us have imagined ourselves superior beings for
most of our lives. For these people, balance can be restored
by going to the opposite extreme for a period of time. Such
people should practice devotional worship of their chosen
divinity. They should also attempt to establish and visualize
the divinity of other beings. The practice of serving others
can also help to restore the balance. It is not by chance that
yogas have developed for each of these techniques. (Devotional yoga is called *Bhakti* Yoga; yoga of service is called
Karma Yoga.) These practices should establish the equality
of all beings.

Others of us have worshiped God, or our chosen divinity,
to the extent that we have made ourselves sinners and inferior
beings. Our rationale is that God is perfect, we are not God,
we are imperfect. Such people must practice seeing the
divinity within themslves. They must recognize that they
are not selves separate from God. They must internalize,
bring back within the fold of their beingness, all of those
aspects of themselves that they have previously cast off by
wrongly thinking they are not divine. *Jnana* Yoga, yoga of
the intellect, and *Raja* Yoga, a composite yoga, are ideal
for this type of person.

In any case, edges must be softened so that they can fade
away naturally and Kundalini can advance unchallenged.
Each man must convince himself that while he is an individual
intellect, while he is an individual mind, while he is an individual body, and while he is an individual soul, he is truly
an individual only in God.

There are a number of "canned" meditations that can help
to restore self-perspective and hasten the advance of the
Kundalini. These meditations are designed to illuminate the
ignorance of ego and to show that recognizing true equality
is the only way to experience the higher being within. Some
time should be set aside each day to dwell on these thoughts.
They are also excellent topics for discussion with your
friends.

Meditation 1: The King, the Beggar, and the Rat

Imagine yourself in a dingy room far from home. Here there are no ties with your previous existence — no loved ones, no friends, no personal belongings.

At once, an arrow pierces your heart, shot through the window from outside. You stand in the center of the room where you begin to slump to the floor in death.

Standing before you is a king in all his regal attire. Beside him is a beggar dressed in rags. And on the other side of the beggar, standing on his hind feet, is a rat. All three have halted their activity and now watch you in your death, as though they all know with certainty that you die.

In that last second, with your eyes still wide from the shock of the blow, meaning comes to you. You look at the others in the room and **see** them for the first and last time in your life. You see that they are really no different from one another. The king and the beggar are basically the same: it no longer makes any sense to bow to one and spit on the other. And the rat — the rat is as important with life as the king and the beggar.

Meditation 2: The Search

What was the last thing you wanted badly? A bike? An automobile? A raise in pay or promotion? Now that you've gotten it, how do you feel about it? Has some of the glitter washed away? What will you want next? And how will you feel about it six months after you get it? Won't you be back where you started?

Man steps from one possession to another. This includes his "spiritual" possessions. Imagine that you can occasionally see the future in your dreams — how long will it be until you want to further expand your psychic capabilities? If you continue to exist under this philosophy, what will happen to you when you "have it all?" Will you be happy?

There is only one thing that man really wants. It manifests and disguises itself in the thousands of other desires he has from day to day. He wants to know who he is. And when he has this knowledge, he needs nothing else.

Try to imagine what it is that would totally satisfy you.

Meditation 3: Bad Versus Good

What is "bad" and what is "good?" Who says so? What does he know?

Couldn't something you believe to be evil actually be a blessing for some other person, or for you at some other time and place, or for some other race of beings, or for some larger aspect of universal survival that you aren't even aware of? With what we now know about how man pollutes his environment, isn't it even possible that man, himself, might be a blight to the larger scale of existence? In this light, might not even the total destruction of man be viewed as "good" to some aspect of the universe?

Who can be the judge of what is bad and what is good?

Why is the search for the unknown sometimes thought of as tampering with the forces of evil?

What is the tree of knowledge of good and evil? Is this "knowledge" an excursion into knowledge or into ignorance? Are not ignorance, illusion and sin all related?

If you can't really tell what is good and what is evil, why should you ever be afraid?

Meditation 4: Ordinary Versus Extraordinary

Who defines a specific object as ordinary or extraordinary? Can something that is extraordinary for one person be ordinary for another? Doesn't the extraordinary always become ordinary with time?

Each man exists at the center of a circle with his collection of things confined with him in the circle. He continually reaches out of the circle to drag new, extraordinary experiences into the circle. When they get there, he no longer wants them. This is man's condition. It is caused by the desire to know self, which manifests as the desire for things. Wouldn't it make more sense for man to try to know self, to wipe out the circle?

And what about spiritual experiences? Are they fundamentally any different from the mundane things we reach for from within our circles? Doesn't everything already belong to the larger self anyway? Who needs it? Come into perspective and know yourself...

There are countless other meditations that you can define

for yourself to help put things into the proper perspective. You can dwell on any of the standard topics of spirituality: love, *maya* (the world of illusion), the nature of relationships and implied contracts with one another, small self versus large self, the nature of divinity, the nature of fear—all of these can help to restore proper perspective and reduce the swelled ego that holds us in ignorance and prevents us from experiencing the Kundalini.

Ramana Maharshi, a great Indian sage, popularized one such meditation. His way of restoring self-perspective was to constantly enquire, "Who am I?" He would then go on to answer himself, "I am not the body, not the mind, not this, not that,—" until all that was left was what he was. This is a very powerful meditation, which, by itself, is the basis of some spiritual practices. According to the texts, it alone can sometimes waken the Kundalini.

Shared Kundalini Experience: Being alone in your experiences and opinions of Kundalini phenomena is initially an obstacle because you stand alone against the standard consensus reality created by the bulk of people around you. This can very quickly sap your psychic strength and bring doubt. On the other hand, surrounding yourself with friends who are also interested in Kundalini-type phenomena can bolster your strength and put some fire into your psychic adventures.

The rational linear thinkers of the world form a collective, agreed-upon reality in which they live comfortably because of the degree of predictability as to what can and cannot happen. We are all caught up in this web, which acts as an invisible, protective barrier to keep us from experiencing some of the stronger, disorienting psychic effects.

Joining forces with other people who are also expanding their belief structures seems to form a new subset of agreed-upon possibilities that permits the more conventional realities to be bypassed on occasion. The synergistic effect of the group forms an oasis of increased possibilities within the desert of time-and space-locked realities we usually accept as normal. Over a period of time, the synergistic effect of *satsang* will pull the entire group toward a psychic level and ability higher than the highest individual in the group. Most, if not all, participants will begin to experience Kundalini effects that were not available to them as lone wolves.

In addition, the other members of the group perform an invaluable service to you by validating your experiences and giving you courage to go on when you need it. Without this service, doubt and fear can very quickly creep into your life to halt the Kundalini process.

Relationships with others who are interested in Kundalini development must be nutured gently and brought along slowly. But once formed, these bonds of friendship and like-thinking will be stronger and more enduring than any you have had before.

To start these relationships, you might introduce some of your more broad-minded friends to some of the more general, yet interesting books related to psychic phemonema. For example, you might introduce them to a book that approaches psychic phenomena from a western, scientific standpoint—perhaps something on the marriage of physics and mysticism. Then, as they read through the revolutionary, "new" ideas in these books, and as their exitement grows, you can engage them in discussions and introduce them to some of the more esoteric Kundalini books. But don't push them too fast.

Soon you will be sharing Kundalini experiences on a day-to-day basis. And your friends will be closer to you than any friends you have had before. After all, each of you will have extended your own being to encompass the others.

There are no specific methods or procedures to engage in with your friends. Just sharing your experiences and your deepest thoughts is more than sufficient. You might occasionally want to experiment with telepathy and other psychic aspects, but treat these as games, and **don't indulge often.** Stay away from **any** formalization of procedure or you will stultify your natural relationships with your friends and reduce the flow of psychic power that moves among you.

In your individual group meditations, practice healing yourself and your friends through right thought. Project love to your friends and accept love from them. Verbally agree to take on some of their suffering or illness during their bad times. (When you do this, expect to **feel** their problems for a short time, yourself.) Give them the same care and love you give yourself.

Put very simply, the more people you can experience this selfless love with, the larger will be your own being.

Formal Practice

The one rule you must remember if you want the Kundalini currents to rise is that you must take the time and effort necessary to come to this state. You must practice what you wish to become! Wishing is only the first phase of attainment: you must then do some work.

We all have a tendency toward a failing in which we **read** about psychic and spiritual practices, but we don't then **do** anything about them. We go on living vicarioiusly without ever acting to bring these things into our lives. You might argue that the books on the subject say that nothing need be done, that we should just live naturally. And this is true, but Western man must first **do** before he can **be.** It is his nature that he must exhaust himself before he can just naturally be.

There are four formal practices I recommend you take up: some form of meditation, chanting, a selection of suitable yogic practices, and biofeedback training to develop your alpha and theta wave generation capabilities. Three of these — meditation, chanting, and practice of yoga — must be practiced **with heart.** If you can't feel them, they are not right for you, and will do you no good. In line with this, the specific selection of meditation, chanting, and yoga techniques must be yours: you must select what feels right to you. The fourth practice, biofeedback, is highly recommended to speed up the Kundalini process. Practice it with **anticipation.**

At first you will probably want to experiment with different types of meditation. This is okay: divide your formal meditation times across these types. Transcendental Meditation or any meditation that uses a mantra is excellent as a basic technique.*

Chanting, by yourself or with a group of people, has an euphoric effect, and is quite powerful in helping to stir the currents and raise the Kundalini. One can chant previously written chants, or one can perform *Japa,* a non-musical repetition of the name of God (*Rama, So Ham, Om Namah Shivaya,* or others). An entire yoga, *Japa* Yoga, is devoted to the practice of devotional verbalization.

* The average Westerner may prefer, for example, the meditation described in H. Benson's *"The Relaxation Response,"* published by William Morrow and Company of New York. This book takes the subjectivity out of meditation and discusses it in scientific terms.

There are scores of yogas to choose from. Each yoga stresses something slightly different from the other yogas. Some yogas appeal to the intellectual person, some to the emotional person; some are designed to prepare the body for the Kundalini experience, others to prepare the mind. Although not common knowledge, **all** yogas, even the Westernized Hatha yoga, have as their esoteric goal the Kundalini experience.

The perspective Kundalini subject will need to invest a good deal of reading time in the various yogas just to familiarize himself with the types that are most suitable for his own specific practice. I recommend starting with books on Kundalini yoga, Integral Yoga, Siddha Yoga, Bhakti Yoga, Raja Yoga, Japa Yoga, Jnana Yoga, and Hatha Yoga for broad, initial coverage of the various types of yoga that are available.

Biofeedback may be **the** key to unlocking the Western door to the Kundalini event. I recommend purchasing a good, medium range, EEG biofeedback unit. As with anything else, you get what you pay for. Expect to pay about $700 dollars for a suitable unit. Much less than this, and you may just as well have saved your money. If the cost is prohibitive, plan to spend some time at an institute in which biofeedback training (EEG) is offered for a reasonable fee.

Remember that biofeedback concentrates the physiological effects of meditation into a shorter time period. You don't want to arouse the Kundalini before you are ready. Use the machine sensibly and your risk will be minimal.

To summarize: Before you begin in earnest, be sure you have the determination to continue. Then let the higher being within you have the reins. Practice becoming a "good" person, not only for the benefit of others, but to protect you from yourself.

Have the courage to stand in the winds of the adverse forces, but do not fight fear, as this will only build its strength. Let your fears dissolve in the knowledge that you are eternal in the one being.

Associate with others like yourself: they will give you needed strength. Be a compassionate and loving warrior and you will see Kundalini bubble forth within you.

PART 4: KUNDALINI WE

SPECULATION ON THE GROWTH OF A COLLECTIVE KUNDALINI

We have become greedy and materialistic in the West. In our drive to more and bigger and better possessions, we have made ourselves smaller and smaller in the important values of life. We have shrunk ourselves into very tight, little knots of individuated consciousness and separated ourselves from that which is all life. And, of course, in doing this, we have turned ourselves into objects—something to be picked up, examined, and then discarded. We have externalized all of our responsibilities toward maintaining ourselves; we have ostracized our own innards.

Instead of seeing wholes, we see parts. Our world is not unified and coherent; it is instead a world of edges and hard objects. Our viewpoint has separated us from the source of life, and now we can no longer see our roots in divinity. And the hurt, the emptiness, the void, is today felt more markedly than ever before.

But natural law will let the process of individuation carry on only so far, and then it will require that the individuated society collapse back into its collective reality, into God.

And this is what we see today. The violence, the thousands of cults that spring into existence and then fade away, the turbulence in our cities—all of this is a scrambling to find our way back to the source. It is the storm that precedes change.

Materialism is both the antithesis and the catalyst for the process of returning to God. What we think is our real destiny—control of nature, possession of all the luxuries of life, a better standard of living—retards our progress toward living in oneness and peace because this goal *turns us into objects.* Yet materialism holds within it the seeds of its own collapse.

The longer we hold out, the more violent will be the return, the collapse into the source. Our situation is like an earthquake: if we can relieve the stress in frequent, little jumps, the effect is not so disruptive. But if we hold out for the big one, all of our walls come crashing down upon us.

We are all involved in the collective influence of the advancing Kundalini in the world today, whether we like it or not. Those who can accept change and adapt to a new, less materially-oriented existence will undergo a minimum of discomfort in the coming years. But the vast multitudes are not ready. They are inundated in materialism and physical comforts.

The coming of the Kundalini, Christ Consciousness, the second coming, salvation, baptism by the Holy Spirit, and the war between Spirituality and Materialism prophesized by some Western Indian tribes are all slightly different views of the same phenomenon: mankind is moving into an age of spirit, an age in which the universe takes a giant, mutational step in its evolutional path.

Before we speculate on Kundalini and the second coming, let's first examine Christ's Kundalini experience, the coming of the dove. For the same kind of experience is available to us all.

Christ and the Kundalini

As did Paul on the road to Damascus, Christ underwent his own personal Kundalini experience. Christ's experience was, however, perhaps the most devastating in recent history. According to the Bible, the event transpired at the time of his baptism by water in the river Jordan. It was followed immediately by confusion, temptation by the Devil, and ministration by God's Angels. (This was during Christ's flight into the wilderness, in which he acclimated himself to the new world.) The onset of the Kundalini experience is indicated in the following passages from the King James version of the Bible, in which John the Baptist tells of seeing the spirit, the light, descend upon Christ at the time of the baptism:

John 1: 32-34. And John bare record, saying, I saw the spirit descending from heaven like a dove, and it abode upon him.

And I knew him not: but he that sent me to baptize with water, the same said unto me, Upon whom thou shalt see the spirit descending, and remaining on him, the same is he which baptizeth with the Holy Ghost.

And I saw, and bare record that this is the Son of God.

Eastern philosophy says that the man who has experienced the Kundalini can, at some point in the cycle, awaken the sleeping Kundalini in others. Swami Muktananda, for example, says that once the Kundalini subject has seen the *blue bindu,* he can "transmit his *Shakti*" (spiritual energy) to others. In Christian tradition, this is Christ's great gift to man: he is a stepping stone to the spirit. In Hindu tradition, this is the gift of Guru to normal man—he brings him from darkness to the light of the spirit. The mechanism is the same.

In the books of Matthew and Mark, Christ himself is said to see the light and hear a voice booming from heaven:

> *Matthew 3:16-17. And Jesus, when he was baptized, went up straightway out of the water: and, lo, the heavens were opened unto him, and he saw the Spirit of God descending like a dove, and lighting upon him:*
> *And lo a voice from heaven saying, This is my beloved Son, in whom I am well pleased.*

The opening of the heavens is a reference to the new universe seen within: heaven is the new state given by the Kundalini experience. During the baptism, Christ's extreme devotional state caused the Kundalini currents to rise within him. The booming voice of God was his own inner thought, magnified to the proportion of a powerful, disincarnate voice.

In the following verses, from the book of Mark, Christ's confusion following the powerful Kundalini experience and the temptation of his banished personality components is told:

> *Mark 1:9-13. And it came to pass in those days, that Jesus came from Nazareth of Galilee, and was baptized of John in Jordan.*
> *And straightway coming up out of the water, he saw the heavens opened, and the Spirit like a dove descending upon him:*
> *And there came a voice from heaven, saying, Thou art my beloved Son, in whom I am well pleased.*
> *And immediately the spirit driveth him into the wilderness.*
> *And he was there in the wilderness forty days, tempted of Satan; and was with the wild beasts; and the angels ministered unto him.*

For forty days and nights, Christ was in a world where all of his inner attitudes, tendencies, emotions and thoughts were played out before him. The Kundalini experience had brought him his own, personal judgement day. This experience must have been a shattering, mind-boggling event. How could it do other than to change his life completely?

Eastern philosophy speaks of the same kind of manifestations in particularly strong Kundalini experiences. It is not uncommon for the subject to see wild beasts, the fires of hell, or angels before him. Neither is it uncommon to hear the voices of powerful, disincarnate beings.

The experience will usually abate within a few hours or days. But for Christ, it took forty days and nights before the currents died down within him. His brain must have been changed radically. He entered his new world to stay.

The light Christ saw was his own internal life's light, invoked by love, devotion, purity, and high emotion, with perhaps a twist of anticipation. The "voice" from heaven was his own thought process, magnified into an intense, audible level. It is possible that it was so intense that it was even experienced in empathy (rhythm entrainment) by John, who was also in a highly emotional state. The temptation was the immediate reaction of Christ's banished mental functions and negative emotions to return to their pre-experience state. As integration of Christ's new personality structure took place, the temptations dwindled, until:

Luke 4:13. And when the devil had ended all the temptation, he departed from him for a season.

The Matthew and Mark versions of the temptation make it clear that both the Devil and God's Angels ministered to Christ. Both Christ's "good" and "bad" aspects had come to the fore: the gates to heaven and hell were side by side.

And as mentioned in the heart of this book, this is what we can all expect to go through, to some degree, after experiencing the Kundalini awakening. We will all see our own tendencies, magnified to gigantic proportions. We can prepare for this by bettering ourselves prior to the experience.

The Bible illustrates that the individual Kundalini event is but the **start** of the spiritual process. While in Christ's case the ego may have died at the time of the event, this will not happen to the majority of us. Each of us will have yet to

experience the full ego death and subsequent resurrection
into a fully enlightened state sometime after the Kundalini
event. The story of Christ illustrates this in the death of Christ
and his subsequent resurrection in God. It further illustrates
a second coming, a final coming, in which the light of God
is brought to all mankind.

Kundalini and the Second Coming

On the second go-round, Glory comes to stay. At this
time, the Son of man and the Son of God become one. In
some cases, according to the Hindus, the body drops away,
no longer needed, and man is home with God. In other cases,
man remains to minister to other men as a *Jivanmukti*, a
liberated man in the flesh.

Christ's first coming was a great gift to mankind. It was a
collective baptism by water. The second coming of the Christ
Consciousness will be on an even grander scale: it will be
a baptism by fire that will catch up all humanity. Those
who have already individually undergone the Kundalini
baptism by fire, which is perhaps a microcosm of the second
coming, will make the transition easily. But those who have
rejected the event will see destruction, chaos, and death
in their material world.

For the second coming will bear a new breed of beings:
a new Son of man, Homo Superior, will appear on the face
of the earth. The earth, itself, will be radically altered. Christ
tells of this in the following account from Luke:

> *Luke 21:6-12. As for these things which ye behold,
> the days will come, in which there shall not be left
> one stone upon another, that shall not be thrown down.*
>
> *And they asked him, saying, Master, but when shall
> these things be? And what sign will there be when
> these things shall come to pass?*
>
> *And he said, Take heed that ye be not deceived:
> for many shall come in my name, saying, I am Christ;
> and the time draweth near: go ye not therefore after
> them.*
>
> *But when ye shall hear of wars and commotions,
> be not terrified: for these things must first come to
> pass; but the end is not by and by.*

Then he said unto them, Nation shall rise against nation, and kingdom against kingdom:

And great earthquakes shall be in diverse places, and famines, and pestilences; and fearful sights and great signs shall there be from heaven.

But before all these, they shall lay their hands on you, and persecute you, delivering you up to the synagogues, and into prisons, being brought before kings and rulers for my name's sake...

Luke 21:20. And when ye shall see Jerusalem compassed with armies, then know that the desolation thereof is nigh.

And then the coming—

Luke 21:25-28. And there shall be signs in the sun, and in the moon, and in the stars; and upon the earth distress of nations, with perplexity; the sea and the waves roaring;

Men's hearts failing them for fear, and for looking after those things which are coming on the earth: for the powers of heaven shall be shaken.

And they shall see the Son of man coming in a cloud with power and great glory.

And when these things begin to come to pass, then look up, and lift up your heads; for your redemption* draweth nigh..

Luke 21:32-36. Verily, I say unto you, This generation shall not pass away, till all be fulfilled.

Heaven and earth shall pass away: but my words shall not pass away.

And take heed to yourselves, lest at any time your hearts be overcharged with surfeiting, and drunkenness, and cares of this life, and so that day come upon you unawares.

For as a snare shall it come on all them that dwell on the face of the whole earth.

Watch ye therefore, and pray always, that ye may be accounted worthy to escape all these things that shall come to pass, and to stand before the Son of man.

---

* A calling back into the God being; a turning in of the old for the new.

A powerful message. And something to think about, whether you believe it or not. Chapter 13 of Mark and Chapter 24 of Matthew contain corresponding accounts of the coming.

From these accounts, and from corresponding signs of the times in evidence today, it can be speculated that Christ had seen precognitively into our age, as have other great beings before and after Christ. And he knew, from his own experiences with the psychic forces generated by the Kundalini currents, that the psychic atmosphere we would generate in our time would rip the very fabric of our material universe. He knew that full control of the force would come very slowly because even he was not in complete control of it, as he implies in John 14:12.

> *Verily, verily, I say unto you, He that believeth on me, the works that I do shall he do also; and greater works than these shall he do; because I go unto my Father.*

Christ knew that the effect would build, collectively, and that the universe, itself, would crumble before us. He knew of the power of God within the Son of man. He knew that while a single spiritual being can cause a wall to crack loudly, many spiritual beings can crack the wall, itself; and a host of spiritual beings can crack a world.

Control of the incredibly powerful Kundalini forces is the root of the prophesized war between Spirituality and Materialism, God and the Devil. It is a war that will be waged within and around each and every one of us.

A Modern Parallel to the Second Coming

In recent years, physics, metaphysics, and religion have all begun to come together. More and more people, religious and non-religious alike, now understand that all paths lead to the same goal: self, knowledge, God.

Subatomic physics, for example, has shown that there may be no "smallest particle," that the universe may in fact be more like a thought than a physical structure. Physics now postulates that all critters of the universe are part of one big bowl of soup: one holographic, inter-dependent, single event that spreads across all time.

In *"Stalking the Wild Pendulum,"* Itzhak Bentov illustrated the holographic unity of the universe by showing how interference patterns record all that goes on. He gave a hypothetical example in which three stones were dropped simultaneously into a bowl of water. The ripples emanating from each of the stones spread out and interacted with one another, producing complex interference patterns in the waves. He went on to explain that if the bowl of water was to be quickfrozen, some strange and amazing records of what had transpired could be obtained. After freezing the ice, one could remove it from the bowl and shine a coherent light (a laser beam) through it. This would cause a holographic, 3-dimensional image of the three stones to be projected into the air somewhere behind the piece of ice.* In other words, the interference patterns would have recorded the event exactly as it occured!

The really startling point of this experiment, however, is that chips of ice can be broken away from the main mass to produce the same effect! That is, when the coherent beam is directed through any of the chips, the same holographic image of the stones, in miniature replica, is projected into the air.

The incredible fact that this reveals is that all that ever happens in the universe is indelibly recorded in the natural interference patterns of reality. All that we see, all that we know, has been molded and recorded by the interference pattern activity that continually shakes the universe into its current form. And the sum total of this information is available in the smallest piece of "matter" in existence. It is all one big event.**

---

* In reality, the ripples returning from the edge of the bowl would distort the image. Actually, the entire event, including the fact that the stones were in a bowl (and that the bowl was in a room, and that the room was in a house, etc.) ,would be recorded in the frozen interference patterns. A practical experiment desirous of seeing a near likeness of the stones would require a very large bowl in which only a small portion of water, immediately surrounding the stones, was quick-frozen.

Or perhaps, one **small event. Bob Toben, in *"Space-Time and Beyond,"* a Dutton Paperback Original, postulates that there may be only one small unit of existence that replicates itself infinitely throughout space and time. In this view, the holographic universe would be constructed from the bottom up, or from small to large, rather than from the top down, large to small.

Bentov further postulates that man's brain is a miniature holographic replica of the workings of the universe, and that man is linked inextricably to the process of reality.

In other words, the universe, with man, is a whole: a self-molding, evolving, "humaeo-universal" organism. And the intellect man has developed gives him a means to superimpose process upon process. Man's intellect is an "external" volition that permits him to consciously control the evolutionary, self-molding process. It forms not only man's body, but the entire universal system.

The question now becomes, How does the rising Kundalini affect this relationship of man and universe?

First, as you have all heard many times, man uses (consciously) only about 1/10 of his brain under normal circumstances. Immediately before the classical Kundalini event and continuing for a while after, the rising Kundalini currents reach into unused portions of the brain where they stimulate the unused cells to a degree never before attained. This increased cellular coverage undoubtedly opens the subject to new sensations, perceptions, and internal experiences that were not available to him prior to the Kundalini experience.

But what is most amazing is that these effects are not restricted to internal physiological manifestations only! The heavy currents in the brain also somehow correspond with the **undoing or redoing of time and space** in a literal sense.

It is not that time and space no longer exist in a perceptive sense (which is perhaps the experience of a truly bicameral man), but the universal cause and effect system itself is somehow distorted so that it is no longer only sequential and linear. Entire sequences of causes and effects are displaced— as in the case of feelies—as reality itself is jostled about.

This means that each person, through his brain, is tightly linked to all of reality. In fact, each person possesses his own individual reality, his own universe, which is maintained collectively with other universes according to consensus rules. The consensus reality is kept within bounds when brain activity is normal, but is disrupted and torn apart when normal brain patterns are "upset" by the accelerating Kundalini currents. During this time, the human being is not only a spectator of the reality around him, but a **creator** of it in the true sense of the word.

To carry this a step further—the classical awakening, in

which the Kundalini currents "spill over" when the brain
is unable to carry the tremendously increased load of electricity, completely shatters time and space. The holographic
unity of the brain with its surrounding universe is modified—
the humaeo-universal system is **mutated.** In some cases the
heavy currents unify and/or short circuit certain right-brain
and left-brain functions that were not previously structured
in this manner. As a result, new perceptions and internal
functions become cameral, as do different points in time and
space in the external environment.

At the same time, other functions normally shared between
brain halves are severed, and become bicameral. Internal
communications are disrupted in this case, while universal
bindings of one sort or another in the external world are
also shattered: "As above, so below."

Over a period of time following the classical awakening,
the brain heals. The severed functions are restored while
the newly unified functions remain unified (the ideal case).

Thus Kundalini provides an evolutionary direction—a
mutational direction—toward a fully-unified functioning of
the two brain halves and a corresponding fully-unified functioning of man and universe. The direction is such that all
universal functions will eventually operate in a fully-con-
scious , fully-aware state.

Needless to say, man is not yet in full conscious control
of the knowledge of how to make or maintain universes.
But he is rapidly approaching this point. And there will
be accidents, chaos, and increasing perplexity until he gets
there.

The time is coming when current patterns of reality will
be cast aside by man, as outdated and cumbersome as the
stone axe is in today's environment. Man will cut his way
across time and space as though they don't exist. He will toy
with probability patterns within his mind and thereby make
dramatic changes to the external world. As he thinks, so it
will be.

Collective, agreed-upon reality will be a thing of the past.
There will be a full, individual universe for each of us as
personal control of individual reality patterns replaces today's
tightly limited consensus reality.

Those who have experienced some of the more profound
distortions of time and space created by the Kundalini effect

understand the nature of the chaos that mankind must soon pass through. They know that as more and more people begin to raise the Kundalini currents, the collective effect will grow, and strange, earth-rocking events will come to pass. They know that the physical laws of the consensus universe, which have already begun to bend, will break, and all of man's artificial constructions will come tumbling down as the collective universe crumbles before him.

For how far a leap is it from making walls crack, seeing into the future, bending forks, disrupting electrical and magnetic flows, and reading minds to producing massive earthquakes and other "natural" disturbances, or to hurling large and ponderous objects through space by the power of will alone?

And as we stumble out of our collective universe into our individual universes, how will we react to the new environment? How will we feel when a wall disappears here and there and a building collapses at our feet, or when a person appears out of nowhere to confront us? How will we react when we realize beyond a doubt that yesterday can be tomorrow, and that the ground is no longer the safe, non-mutable substance beneath our feet that it once was? How will we react to the white light permeating the expansive night sky from horizon to horizon; Jesus Christ returned on his white steed; unidentified flying objects popping into and out of existence in ever increasing numbers?

It will take some getting used to.

But eventually, we will emerge from this period of confusion and perplexity. And from our new-found individualism we will form a new collective universe—one in which "sorcery" and "magic" will be the new natural law; one in which the spiritual man, the meek, will live in peace with himself and with other men, for those of other nature will be no more.

The age of the Kundalini man is dawning.

APPENDIX AND BIBLIOGRAPHY

Appendix A: Biofeedback and Kundalini Arousal

Biofeedback is a recent scientific development that provides a means for man to monitor and control the activity of body functions not normally associated with conscious volition. It is an application of the engineering servo-mechanism principle used to control automatic machine functions. For example, a furnace and a thermostat form a **feedback** system that controls the temperature of the house. With this arrangement, the temperature of the house is, itself, the information that is **fed back** to the thermostat. When the thermostat senses that the temperature has gone above or below the acceptable range, it "tells" the furnace what to do. In this manner, the furnace and the thermostat work together to regulate the temperature.

Normally, such a system is set to certain preselected system parameters. These parameters are established by a volition that is external to the servomechanistic unit, itself. In the case of the furnace and the thermostat, **man** is the volition. He adjusts the setting to establish the range in which he wants the unit to operate.

A **biofeedback** system is a feedback system in which biological activity is sensed, firsthand, and thereby fed back to the biological organism (man) who is both the source and the sensor of his own internal, physiological activity. With biofeedback, man inserts himself into a servomechanistic loop. He becomes both the furnace and the volition. Selected body conditions are monitored by the biofeedback machine, the thermostat. Effectively, the biofeedback machine becomes the eyes of man's own internal, physiological functions.

By seeing and hearing this feedback information firsthand, the biofeedback subject learns how to control body functions that would not normally be under his conscious control. And so, using his volition, he can then change the system parameters at will, just as he changes the thermostat setting.

The fact that man can learn to control body responses that were previously thought to be autonomic has caused a great deal of excitement in scientific and medical ranks. And in the late 1960's biofeedback began to gain a great deal of medical respectability. Today it is used in a host of medical and theraputic applications such as:

- Controlling migraine headaches
- Assisting in paralysis recovery
- Providing relief from stress
- Controlling the blood pressure
- Reducing the severity and frequency of epileptic seizures
- Providing gastrointestinal control
- Relaxing the muscles
- Assisting in motor training
- Reinforcing the physiological effects of meditation

and many others. It has even been used, experimentally, to control functional diarrhea and penile tumescence!

There are three major classifications of biofeedback devices: skin temperature monitoring devices, electromyography (EMG) machines, and electroencephalography (EEG) machines. Most, if not all, of these machines are simply variations of existing medical monitoring devices that permit the person who is being monitored to sense, and thereby control, his own output.

Skin Temperature Monitoring Devices: These devices can be used in various medical applications. One major use for this type of device is to help control migraine headaches. In such a usage, temperature sensing probes are attached to the patient's hands. The patient is told that the audible tone produced by the monitor indicates how hot his hands are — the higher the tone, the hotter the hands. If he can raise the tone of the machine, he is told, he will also be raising the temperature of his hands. This will head off his headaches.

And it works! For some reason, raising the hand temperature heads off migraine headaches in a large percentage of people who suffer from migraines. What's more, having seen how he can control his hand temperature with the machine, the patient soon learns the "feel" of how to do this without the machine. Then he can apply this feel to his daily life whenever he thinks a migraine headache is about to strike.

EMG Devices: These devices are used to monitor muscular conditions. In one such application, the EMG device is used to teach the patient how to relax his muscles and lessen the tension in his body. A typical use measures the muscle tension of the frontalis muscle in the forehead. An audible note indicates the degree of tension in this muscle. The patient is instructed to lower the tone to relax the forehead muscle. When he can successfully do this, the remainder of the major muscles in his body seem to follow the lead of the frontalis muscle. As with the skin temperature monitoring devices, the subject soon gets the feel of how to do this. He can then apply the technique in his daily life without the machine.

EEG Devices: The EEG device is the one we are most concerned with as an aid to awakening the Kundalini. This device monitors brain waves, electrical discharges by the neurons in the brain.

The neurons can "fire," or discharge, at a rate between one cycle and thirty cycles per second (CPS). Usually, the higher rates indicate that the subject is in a state of mental attention: the neurons are firing asynchronously. As the subject relaxes his thoughts and lets go, the frequency begins to get lower as the neurons begin to fire synchronously. Because the outputs of the individual neurons reinforce one another at this time, the strength, or amplitude, of the brainwaves increases. Time spent in this lower frequency/higher amplitude state brings on bliss and reinforces the meditative state.

Research has indicated that certain ranges of frequencies correlate roughly to focused attention, relaxed awareness, creativity, and deep meditation. The EEG device can be used to inform the subject as to which range of frequencies he is currently generating. Through various tones, metering, and visual indicators on the machine, the subject can learn how to enter the various ranges of frequencies at will. In this way, he can train himself to establish the mental environment in which these subjective states seem to flourish. The nomenclature and frequencies assicated with these four states follow:

Brainwave State	Frequency (CPS)	Subjective State
Beta	13 and up	Focused concentration
Alpha	8 to 12	Relaxed awareness
Theta	4 to 7	Creativity; visual imagery; emotional peaks
Delta	0+ to 3	Deep sleep; deep meditation

In about four hours of machine time, one can learn to generate alpha range frequencies at many spots on the head. With more practice, the theta range, with its accompanying visions and creative states, can be reached. Some subjects can learn to produce delta range frequencies even while remaining awake—a most difficult task. All of this training quickens the arrival of the Kundalini.

Any subject dealing with man's brain is, of course, highly complex. As such, the descriptions and explanations of biofeedback have been given a broadbrush treatment in this volume. There are a number of good commercial publications on the subject of biofeedback available at your local book store. One or two of these should bring you up to speed before you begin to think of purchasing a specific biofeedback machine. For the more serious student of biofeedback, I recommend a series of medical and general papers on biofeedback compiled by the Aldine Publishing Company of Chicago. This series provides all of the important developments in biofeedback since 1969, and is titled *"Biofeedback and Self-Control: An Aldine Annual on the Regulation of Bodily Processes and Consciousness."*

I would also recommend a good book on the geography of various brain functions, a subject unto itself. One that comes to mind is *"Speech and Brain-Mechanisms,"* by Wilder Penfield and Lamar Roberts, published by Atheneum, New York.

One last caution about the use of biofeedback as a means to raise the Kundalini: it is still uncharted territory to a large degree. It is a form of mountain climbing in that there is a very real element of danger mixed with the promise of fulfillment that would not be achieved by a more normal pursuit of life. The outcome of extensive time on the biofeedback machine cannot be accurately predicted.

Remember that while you experience pleasant highs, and while you reap the psychic fruits, you are modifying the way your brain works—a ticklish situation. I would urge you to proceed cautiously, or you might get there before you are ready.

There are many surprises in store for you—some you will like, some you will not like. But then again, if you never know who you are, what good is it?

Bibliography

Books and Authors Referred to:

The Bible, King James Version

Benson, H. *The Relaxation Response*, William Morrow and Company

Bentov, I. *Stalking the Wild Pendulum*, Dutton

Biofeedback and Self-Control: An Aldine Annual on the Regulation of Bodily Processes and Consciousness, Aldine

Bucke, R. M. *Cosmic Consciousness*, Dutton

Castenada, Carlos. General reference to his series of Don Juan books

Chaney, Earlyne. *Remembering: The Autobiography of a Mystic*, Astara/New Age Press

Jones, Franklin. *Knee of Listening*, Dawn Horse Press

Krishna, Gopi. *The Evolutionary Energy in Man*, Shambhala

Muktananda, Swami. *Sadgurunath Maharaj Ki Jay*, c/o G.P.O. Box 1718, New York, N.Y. 10001

Penfield, Wilder and Lamar Roberts. *Speech and Brain-Mechanisms*, Atheneum

Roberts, Jane. *Seth Speaks*, Prentice-Hall

Sannella, Lee. *Kundalini: Psychosis or Transcendence*, H. Dakin, San Francisco

Satprem. *Sri Aurobindo, or the Adventure of Consciousness*, Harper and Row

Toben, Bob. *Space-Time and Beyond*, Dutton

Acknowledgements to Julian Jaynes for introducing me to the term "bicameral," which I first saw in reviews of his book, *"The Origins of Consciousness in the Breakdown of the Bicameral Mind."*

Suggested Books on Dreams:

Crisp, Tony. *Do You Dream*, Dutton

Faraday, Ann. *Dream Power*, Berkly Medallion; *The Dream Game*, Harper and Row

Fodor, Nandor. *Dream Interpretation*, Citadel Press

Garfield, P. *Creative Dreaming*, Simon and Schuster

Green, Celia. *Lucid Dreams*, Hamish Hamilton, London

Holzer, Hans. *The Psychic Side of Dreams*, Doubleday

Jung, C.G. *Man and His Symbols*, Dell

Stekel, Wilhelm. *The Interpretation of Dreams*, Liveright

Ullman, M., S. Krippner, A. Vaughan. *Dream Telepathy*, Penguin

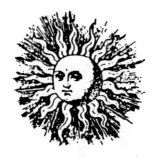

OTHER SUN BOOKS TITLES

you may find of interest:

ASTROLOGY

ALAN LEO'S DICTIONARY OF ASTROLOGY by Alan Leo and Vivian E. Robson. Aaron's Rod, Casting the Horoscope, Disposition, Ecliptic, Equinoxes, Period of Sun, Objects Governed by the Planets, Mean Time.

THE ASTROLOGICAL GUIDE TO HEALTH FOR EACH OF THE TWELVE SUN SIGNS by Ariel Gordon, M.C. Information regarding the twelve signs of the Zodiac is taken from seven of the greatest authorities, past and present, on the different correspondences, as well as from personal experience, extending over many years of private practice.

ASTROLOGICAL PREDICTION by P.J. Harwood. Studing Astrology, Place and Time in Different Parts of the World, Erecting Horoscopes, Astrological Predictions, Definitions of Terms and Abbreviations, Transits and Various Directions, Life Periods, The Radical Horoscope, Marriage, Travel, Change and General Fortune, Time of Action, How Knowing Directions can Influence the Course of Life, Horoscopical Studies of Famous Individuals.

ASTROLOGY: HOW TO MAKE AND READ YOUR OWN HOROSCOPE by Sepharial. The Alphabet of the Heavens, The Construction of a Horoscope, How to Read the Horoscope, The Stars in Their Courses.

A BEGINNER'S GUIDE TO PRACTICAL ASTROLOGY by Vivian E. Robson. How to Cast a Horoscope, Planets, Signs, and Houses, How to Judge a Horoscope, How to Calculate Future Influences, etc.

THE BOWL OF HEAVEN by Evangeline Adams. My Job and How I Do It, A Grim Success, A Tale of Two Cities, "Dabbling in Heathenism", A Horrible Example, We are All Children of the Stars, Life and Death, The Money-Makers, Some Ladies of Venus, I Never Gamble, A World in Love, Astrological Marriages, My Own and Others, The New Natology, Twins and Things, Why Most People Come to Me, Am I Always Right? As I See It.

THE COSMIC KEY OF LIFE SELF-REALIZATION by A.S. Vickers. Index Charts, The Cosmic Key of Life, Helps in Selecting a Goal, Concentration, What is a Science? Key to Horoscope Blanks, Horoscopes of Noted Persons, Planetary Positions, Planetary Aspects, Sign Keywords, Appendix To Students, Astrological Smiles, Index to Astrological Attributes.

THE DIVINE LANGUAGE OF CELESTIAL CORRESPONDENCES by Coulson Turnbull. Esoteric Symbolism of the Planets, Mystical Interpretation of the Zodiac, Kabalistical Interpretation of the 12 Houses, Evolution and Involution of Soul, Character of the Planets, Hermetic Books, Nature of Signs, Etc.

THE EARTH IN THE HEAVENS - RULING DEGREES OF CITIES - HOW TO FIND AND USE THEM by L. Edward Johndro. Precession, Midheavens and Ascendants, Calculating Midheavens and Ascendants, Use of Locality Angles, Verification by World Events, Applications to Nativities.

ECLIPSES IN THEORY AND PRACTICE by Sepharial. The Natural Cause of an Eclipse, Eclipses of the Sun, Lunar Eclipses, Historical Eclipses, To Calculate an Eclipse of the Sun, To Calculate a Lunar Eclipse, Eclipse Signs, Eclipse Indications, The Decanates, Transits over Eclipse Points, Individuals and Eclipses, Illustrations, Conclusion.

HEBREW ASTROLOGY by Sepharial. Chaldean Astronomy, Time and Its Measures, The Great Year, The Signs of the Zodiac, How to Set a Horoscope, The Seven Times, Modern Predictions.

THE INFLUENCE OF THE ZODIAC UPON HUMAN LIFE by Eleanor Kirk. The Quickening Spirit, Questions and Answers, Disease, Development, A Warning, Marriage, The Fire, Air, Earth, and Water Triplicities, Etc. (This is an excellent book!)

THE LIGHT OF EGYPT or THE SCIENCE OF THE SOUL AND THE STARS by Thomas H. Burgoyne. Vol. 1: Realms of Spirit and Matter, Mysteries of Sex, Incarnation and Re-Incarnation, Karma, Mediumship, Soul Knowledge, Mortality and Immortality. Basic Principles of Celestial Science, Stellar Influence on Humanity, Alchemical Nature of Man, Union of Soul and Stars. Vol. II: The Zodiac and the Constellations, Spiritual Interpretation of the Zodiac, Astro-Theology and Astro-Mythology, Symbolism and Alchemy, Talismans and Ceremonial Magic, Tablets of AEth including: The Twelve Mansions, The Ten Planetary Rulers, The Ten Great Powers of the Universe, and Penetralia – The Secret of the Soul.

MANUAL OF ASTROLOGY by Sepharial. Language of the Heavens, Divisions of the Zodiac, Planets, Houses, Aspects, Calculation of the Horoscope, Reading of a Horoscope, Measure of Time, Law of Sex, Hindu Astrology, Progressive Horoscope, Etc.

MEDICAL ASTROLOGY by Henrich Däath. Basic Elements, Anatomical Sign-Rulership, Planetary Powers and Principles, Biodynamic Actions of Planets, How the Planets Crystallise in Organic and Inorganic Life, Tonicity, Atonicity and Perversion, Zodiaco-Planetary Synopsis of Typical Diseases, The Sixth and Eight Houses, The Triplicities and Quadruplicities, Planetary Sympathy and Antipathy, Guaging Planetary Strengths in the Specific Horoscope, Application, Examples, Indications of Short Life

NEW DICTIONARY OF ASTROLOGY In Which All Technical and Abstruse Terms Used In The Text Books of the Science Are Intimately Explained And Illustrated by Sepharial. Everything from Abscission to Zuriel.

THE PLANETS THROUGH THE SIGNS: Astrology for Living, by Abbe Bassett. Includes chapters on the Sun, Moon, and various planets, and how each one influences us through the different signs of the Zodiac.

PRIMARY DIRECTIONS MADE EASY by Sepharial. Principles of Directing, Polar Elevations, Illustrations, Mundane Aspects, Zodiacal Parallels, Mundane Parallels, Summary, Further Examples, Suggested Method, General Review, The Royal Horoscope, The Telescopic View, Solar and Lunar Horoscopes, Appendix.

RAPHAEL'S GUIDE TO ASTROLOGY by Raphael. The Symbols Explained, The Nature of the Aspects and Signs, The Orbits of the Planets, Persons Produced by the Signs of The Zodiac, The Form of Body Given by the Planets in the Signs, The Use of an Ephemeris, How to Erect a Map of the Heavens, How to Place the Planets in the Map, The Nature of the Planets, How to Judge a Nativity, Whether a Child Will Live or Die, Health, Mental Qualities, Money, Employment, Marriage, Travel, Etc., On the Selection of a House, Friends and Enemies, Directions or Calculating Future Events, A Short Astrological Dictionary, Etc!

RAPHAEL'S KEY TO ASTROLOGY by Raphael. Planetary Aspects and Orbs, Description of Persons Produced by the Signs, The Use of an Ephemeris, How to Erect a Map of the Heavens, The Influence of the Planets, How to Judge a Nativity, Whether a Child Will Live or Die, Health and Mental Qualities, Money Prospects and Employment, Marriage, Children and Travel, Friends and Enemies, The Kind of Death, etc.

RAPHAEL'S MEDICAL ASTROLOGY or the Effects of the Planets on the Human Body by Raphael. The Zodiac and the Human Body, Planetary Rulership and Action, Health and Constitution, Physical Condition, The Duration of Life, Examples of Early Death, Diseases, Mental Disorders, Injuries, Accidents and Deformities, Health and the Horoscope, Preventive Measures, Herbal Remedies, the Course of Disease, Astrology and Colors, etc.

RAPHAEL'S MUNDANE ASTROLOGY or The Effects of the Planets and Signs Upon the Nations and Countries of the World by Raphael. Mundane Astrology, Planetary and Zodiacal Signs and Symbols, The Twelve Mundane Houses, The Significations of the Planets,

Essential and Accidental Dignities, The Mundane Map, Concerning the Houses and the Planets, How to Judge a Mundane Map, Ellipses, Earthquakes, Comets, Planetary Conjunctions, The Parts of the World Affected by the Signs of the Zodiac. etc.

RELATION OF THE MINERAL SALTS OF THE BODY TO THE SIGNS OF THE ZODIAC by Dr. George W. Carey. Biochemistry, Esoteric Chemistry, The Ultimate of Biochemistry, The Twelve Cell-Salts of the Zodiac, Aries: The Lamb of God, Taurus: The Winged Bull, The Chemistry of Gemini, Cancer: The Chemistry of the Crab, Leo: The Heart of the Zodiac, Virgo: The Virgin Mary, Libra: The Loins, Scorpio: Influence of the Blood, The Chemistry of Sagittarius, Capricorn: The Goat of the Zodiac, The Sign of the Son of Man: Aquarius, Pisces: The Fish That Swim in the Pure Sea.

THE RISING ZODIACAL SIGN: ITS MEANING AND PROGNOSTICS by Coulson Turnbull. Aries - The Ram, Taurus - The Bull, Gemini - The Twins, Cancer - The Crab, Leo - The Lion, Virgo - The Virgin, Libra - The Balance, Scorpio - The Scorpion, Sagittarius - The Arrow, Capricorn - The Goat, Aquarius - The Waterman, Pisces - The Fishes, How To Determine the Rising Sign, Tables I, II, and III.

THE SCIENCE OF FOREKNOWLEDGE AND THE RADIX SYSTEM by Sepharial. The Science of Foreknowledge, Astrology in Shakespeare, The Great Year, Celestial Dynamics, Neptune, The Astrology of Lilith, Indian Astrology, Horoscope of Rama, Astrology of The Hebrews, Joan of Arc, The Measure of Life, Astrological Practice, Methods of Ptolemy and Benatti, The Radix System, Horoscopical Anomalies, Our Solar System, Financial Astrology.

THE SILVER KEY: A GUIDE TO SPECULATIORS by Sepharial. The Furure Method, Science of Numbers, Finding the Winner, The Lunar Key, Gravity and Evolution, Something to Come, A Warning, On Specilation, Monte Carlo and Astrology, Tables of Sidereal Times, Tables of Ascendants, Etc!

THE SOLAR EPOCH A NEW ASTROLOGICAL THESIS by Sepharial. The History of Birth, The Lunar Horoscope, The Solar Horoscope, Directional Influences, Conclusions.

THE SOLAR LOGOS OR STUDIES IN ARCANE MYSTICISM BY Coulson Turnbull. The Logos, The Kingdom of the Soul, Intuition and Motion, The Mystic Macrocosm, The Spirit of the Planets, The Mystical Sun and Moon, The Soul in Action, The Spiritual Horoscope, Health, Disease, Service, Etc.

THE STARS - HOW AND WHERE THEY INFLUENCE by L. Edward Johndro. Theory, Astronomical Fundamentals, Application of Fixed Stars to Nativities, Application of fixed Stars to Mundane Astrology, Verification by Nativities, Verification by World Events, Variable Stars, Binary Stars, Double Stars, Clusters, Nebulae and Bright Stars, General and Technical, Considerations, Conclusion.

STARS OF DESTINY – THE ANCIENT SCIENCE OF ASTROLOGY AND HOW TO MAKE USE OF IT TODAY by Katherine Taylor Craig. History and description of the Science, The Sun From Two Standpoints, The Moon and the Planets. Astrological Predictions That Have Been Verified, Practical Directions for Casting a Horoscope, Sample of General Prediction for a Year.

A STUDENTS' TEXT-BOOK OF ASTROLOGY by Vivian E. Robson. Fundamental Principles of Astrology, Casting the Horoscope, Character and Mind, Occupation and Position, Parents, Relatives and Home, Love and Marriage, Esoteric Astrology, Adoption of the New Style Calendar.

WHAT IS ASTROLOGY? by Colin Bennett. How an Astrologer Works, Sign Meanings, How Aspects Affect a Horoscope, Numerology as an Astrological Aid, Psychology In Relation to Astrology, Etc.

ATLANTIS / LEMURIA

ATLANTIS IN AMERICA by Lewis Spence. Atlantis and Antillia, Cro-Magnons of America. Quetzalcoatl the Atlantean, Atlantis in American Tradition and Religion, Ethnological Evidence, Art and Architecture, Folk-Memories of an Atlantic Continent, Analogy of Lemuria, Chronological Table, Etc.

THE PROBLEM OF LEMURIA - THE SUNKEN CONTINENT OF THE PACIFIC by Lewis Spence, Illustrated. The Legend of Lemuria, The Argument From Archaeology, The Testimony of Tradition, The Evidence from Myth and Magic, The Races of Lemuria, The Testimony of Custom, The Proof of Art, The Geology of Lemuria,

The Evidence from Biology, The Catastrophe and its Results, Life and Civilization in Lemuria, Atlantis and Lemuria, Conclusions.

WISDOM FROM ATLANTIS by Ruth B. Drown. Being, Divine Selfishness, Service, Nobility of Self-Reliance, Harmony, Divine Love, Principles of Life and Living, Man's Divine Nature, Faith, True Thinking.

AUTOSUGGESTION / HYPNOTISM

AUTO-SUGGESTION: WHAT IT IS AND HOW TO USE IT FOR HEALTH, HAPPINESS AND SUCCESS by Herbert A. Parkvn. M.D.. C.M. Auto-suggestion - What it is and how to use it, Auto-suggestion - Its effects and how to employ it to overcome physical troubles, Auto-suggestion - How to employ it to overcome mental troubles, Influences of early auto-suggestions for the forming of the character, Auto-suggestion for the formation of habits, Auto-suggestion and personal magnetism, The cultivation of optimism through auto-suggestion, Auto-suggestion for developing concentration, The achievement of success through auto-suggestion and success, Auto-suggestion and breathing exercises, Auto-suggestion: It's influence on health in the winter, The diagnosis and treatment of a typical case of chronic physical suffering, Auto-suggestion the basis of all healing, How psychic pictures are made realities by auto-suggestion.

EMILE COUÉ: THE MAN AND HIS WORK by Hugh MacNaughten Foreword and Author's Notes, Prelude, Nancy, Nancy or London, M Coué at Eton, M Coué in London, The Sub-Concious Self, On Some Stumbling Blocks, M Coué in His Relation To Christianity, On "Everything for Nothing", M. Coué, Envoi.

HOW TO PRACTICE SUGGESTION AND AUTOSUGGESTION by Emile Coué, Preface by Charles Baudouin. Interviews of Patients, Examples of the Power of Suggestion and Autosuggestion, Suggestions: General and Special, Special Suggestions for Each Ailment, Advice to Patients, Lectures Delivered by Emile Coué in America.

MY METHOD by Emile Coué. Chapters Include: Autosuggestion Disconcerting in its Simplicity, Slaves of Suggestion and Masters of Ourselves, Dominance of the Imagination over the Will, The Moral Factor in all Disease, Don't Concentrate, How to Banish Pain, Psychic Culture as Necessary as Physical, Self-Mastery Means Health, Etc.

THE PRACTICE OF AUTOSUGGESTION BY THE METHOD OF EMILE COUÉ by C. Harry Brooks. The Clinic of Emile Coué, A Few of Coué's Cures, Thought is a Force, Thought and the Will, The General Formula, How to Deal With Pain, Autosuggestion and the Child, Particular Suggestions, Etc.

SELF MASTERY THROUGH CONSCIOUS AUTOSUGGESTION by Emile Coué. Self Mastery Through Autosuggestion, Thoughts and Precepts, What Autosuggestion Can Do, Education as it Ought to Be, A Survey of the "Seances", the Miracle Within, Everything for Everyone, Etc.

SUGGESTION AND AUTOSUGGESTION by Charles Baudouin. Why Do We Ignore Autosuggestion?, Representative Suggestions, Affective Suggestions, Motor Suggestions, Conditional Suggestions, The Action of Sleep, The Law of Reversed Effort, Relaxation and Collectedness, Autohypnosis, Moral Energy, Exercises, Coue's Practice, Acceptivity and Suggestibility, The Education of Children, Methods of Application,

CLAIRVOYANCE

SECOND SIGHT - A STUDY OF NATURAL AND INDUCED CLAIRVOYANCE by Sepharial. The Scientific Position, Materials and Conditions, The Faculty of Seership, Preliminaries and Practice, Kinds of Visions, Obstacles and Clairvoyance, Symbolism, Allied Psychic Phases, Experience and Use.

CONSPIRACY

THE ILLUMINOIDS – SECRET SOCIETIES AND POLITICAL PARANOIA by Neal Wilgus. Detailed picture of Weishaupt's Order of the Illuminati as well as other secret societies throughout history. Ties various far-reaching areas together including important information relating to the J.F. Kennedy assassination. "The best single reference on the Illuminati in fact and legendry" – Robert Anton Wilson in Cosmic Trigger.

CRYSTALS/MINERALS

CRYSTALS AND THEIR USE—A Study of At-One-Ment with the Mineral Kingdom by Page Bryant. Mineral Consciousness, Crystals and Their Use, Sacred Centers, Various Types of Crystals, The Amethyst, Crystal Gazing.

THE MAGIC OF MINERALS by Page Bryant. The Inner Lives of the Mineral Kingdom, Megalithic Mysteries and the Native American View, The Healing Properties of Minerals, Psychic Influences in Minerals, Stones of the Zodiac, Crystals and Their Use, General Information on Selection, Use, and Care of Minerals.

MAN, MINERALS, AND MASTERS by Charles W. Littlefield, M.D. School of the Magi, Three Masters, The Cubes, Initiation in Tibet, Hindustan, and Egypt, History, Prophecy, Numerology, Perfection. 172p. 5x8 Paperback.

PLANETARY INFLUENCES AND THERAPEUTIC USES OF PRECIOUS STONES by George Frederick Kunz. Includes various lists and illustrations, etc.

DREAMS

DREAMS AND PREMONITIONS by L.W. Rogers. Introduction, The Dreamer, The Materialistic Hypotheses Inadequate, Dreams of Discovery, Varieties of Dreams, Memories of Astral Experiences, Help from the Invisibles, Premonitory Dreams, Dreams of the Dead, How to Remember Dreams.

EARTH CHANGES (Also See Prophecy)

CHEIRO'S WORLD PREDICTIONS by Cheiro. Fate of Nations, British Empire in its World Aspect, Destiny of the United States, Future of the Jews, Coming War of Wars, Coming Aquarian Age, Precession of the Equinoxes.

THE COMING STAR-SHIFT AND MANY PROPHECIES OF BIBLE AND PYRAMID FUL-FILLED by O. Gordon Pickett. God Corrects His Clock in the Stars, English Alphabet as Related to Numerics, Joseph Builder of the Great Pyramid, Numerical Harmony, Prophecy, World Wars, Star-Shifts, The Flood, Astronomy, The Great Pyramids, Etc.

COMING WORLD CHANGES by H.A. and F.H.Curtiss. The Prophecies, Geological Considerations, The Philosophy of Planetary Changes, The King of the World, The Heart of the World, The Battle of Armageddon, The Remedy.

EARTH CHANGES NOW! by Page Bryant. The Earth is Changing: The Evidence, We Knew it was Coming!, The Sacred Covenant, The Externalization of the Spiritual Hierarchy, The Earth Angel: A Promise for the Future.

THE EARTH CHANGES SURVIVAL HANDBOOK by Page Bryant. The Emergence of Planetary Intelligence, Mapping the Earth, Earth Changes: Past and Future, Preparing for the Future, Walking in Balance, Etc.

NOSTRADAMUS NOW - PROPHECIES OF PERIL AND PROMISE FOR THE 1990'S AND BEYOND by Joseph Robert Jochmans Chapters include: What Were the Prophet's Secret Sources of Wisdom? What Mysterious Methods Did the Prophet Use to Make His Forecasts? Will the Prophet Return to Life? A Warning of Coming Global War For Our World Today? Is America About to Suffer Social, Political and Economic Collapse? Will Superquakes Devastate America's West and East Coasts? Is a Planetary Inter-Dimensional Doorway About to Be Opened? The Middle East Gulf War Was It Necessary, and Will It Flare Up Again? The Coming of the Man of Power From the East: Antichrist or Avatar? When Will the Downfall of the World Economic System Take Place? Could a Comet or Meteor Hit the Earth and Cause an Axis Pole Shift? Where Will be the Trouble Spots in the Middle East and Far East During the Next Ten Years? What Major Earth Cataclysms May Yet Occur? The New Russia and America Have They Changed For the Better? What Will Be Humanity's Destiny Into the Far Future? Which Future Options Will We Choose?

ORACLES OF NOSTRADAMUS by Charles A. Ward. Life of Nostradamus, Preface to Prophecies, Epistle to Henry II, Magic, Historic Fragments, Etc.

PROPHECIES OF GREAT WORLD CHANGES compiled by George B. Brownell. World-War Prophecies, Coming Changes of Great Magnitude, False Christs, The New Heaven and the New Earth, The New Order and the Old, Etc.

ROLLING THUNDER: THE COMING EARTH CHANGES by J. R. Jochmans. The Coming Famine and Earth Movements, The Destruction of California and New York, Future War, Nostradamus, Bible, Edgar Cayce, Coming Avatars, Pyramid Prophecy, Weather, Coming False Religion and the Antichrist, and much, much more! This book is currently our best selling title.

UTOPIA II: AN INVESTIGATION INTO THE KINGDOM OF GOD by John Schmidt. Why Utopia?, Mankind's Past, Present, and Future, A Sociological Look, A Political Look, An Economic Look, A Spiritual Look.

GENERAL METAPHYSICAL

THE CABALA - ITS INFLUENCE ON JUDAISM AND CHRISTIANITY by Bernard Pick. Name and Origin of the Cabala, The Development of the Cabala in the Pre-Zohar Period, The Book of Zohar or Splendor, The Cabala in the Post Zohar Period, The Most Important Doctrines of the Cabala, The Cabala in Relation to Judaism and Christianity.

THE ESSENES AND THE KABBAIAH Two Essays by Christian D. Ginsburg. Description of the Essenes, Ancient and Modern Literature, The Meaning of the Kabbalah, Kabbalistic Cosmogony, Creation of Angels and Men, The Destiny of Man and the Universe, Kabbalism, the Old Testament, and Christianity, The Books of the Kabbalah, The Schools, Indexes and Glossary.

GEMS OF MYSTICISM by H.A. and F.H. Curtiss. Spiritual Growth, Duty, Karma, Reincarnation, The Christ, Masters of Wisdom.

THE HISTORY AND POWER OF MIND by Richard Ingalese. Divine Mind; It's Nature and Manifestation, Dual Mind and its Origin, Self-Control Re-Embodiment, Colors of Thought Vibration, Meditation, Creation, and Concentration, Psychic Forces and their Dangers, Spiritual Forces and Their Uses, The Cause and Cure of Disease, The Law Of Opulance.

INFINITE POSSIBILITIES by Leilah Wendell. Chapters include: The Essence of Time, Time and Space, Inseperable Brothers, Coexistent Time, Traveling Through Time, Microcosmic Reflections, Cosmic Consciousness, The Universe in a Jar, Psychic Alchemy, Universality, The Divine Element, The Complete Whole, What Price Immortality?, Practical Infinity, Etc.

VISUALIZATION AND CONCENTRATION AND HOW TO CHOOSE A CAREER by Fenwicke L. Holmes. The Creative Power of Mind, Metaphysics and Psychology, Mental Telepathy, Visualization and Dramatization, Concentration How to Choose a Career.

GENERAL OCCULT

THE BOOK OF CHARMS AND TALISMANS by Sepharial. History and Background, Numbers and their Significance, Charms to Wear, Background of Talismans, Making Talismans.

BYGONE BELIEFS – AN EXCURSION INTO THE OCCULT AND ALCHEMICAL NATURE OF MAN by H. Stanley Redgrove. Some Characteristics of Mediaeval Thought, Pythagoras and his Philosophy, Medicine and Magic, Belief in Talismans, Ceremonial Magic in Theory and Practice, Architectural Symbolism, Philosopher's Stone, The Phallic Element in Alchemical Doctrine, Roger Bacon, Etc. (Many Illustrations).

THE COILED SERPENT by C.J. van Vliet. A Philosophy of Conservation and Transmutation of Reproductive Energy. Deadlock in Human Evolution, Spirit Versus Matter, Sex Principle and Purpose of Sex, Pleasure Principle, Unfolding of Spirit, Marriage and Soul-Mates, Love Versus Sex, Erotic Dreams, Perversion and Normalcy, Virility, Health, and Disease, Freemasonry, Rosicrucians, Alchemy, Astrology, Theosophy, Magic, Yoga, Occultism, Path of Perfection, Uncoiling the Serpent, The Future, Supermen, Immortality, Etc.

COSMIC SYMBOLISM by Sepharial. Meaning and Purpose of Occultism, Cosmic Symbology, Reading the Symbols, Law of Cycles, Time Factor in Kabalism, Involution and Evolution, Planetary Numbers, Sounds, Hours, Celestial Magnetic Polarities, Law of Vibrations, Lunar and Solar Influences, Astrology and the Law of Sex, Character and Environment, Etc.

THE ELEUSINIAN MYSTERIES AND RITES by Dudley Wright. Preface, Introduction, The Eleusinian Legend, The Ritual of the Mysteries, Program of the Greater Mysteries, The Intimate Rites, The Mystical Significance, Bibliography.

THE INNER GOVERNMENT OF THE WORLD by Annie Besant. Ishvara, The Builders of a

Cosmos, The Hierarchy of our World, The Rulers, Teachers, Forces, Method of Evolution, Races and Sub-Races, The Divine Plan, Religions and Civilizations, Etc.

THE MASCULINE CROSS AND ANCIENT SEX WORSHIP by Sha Rocco. Origin of the Cross, Emblems: Phallus, Triad, Vocabulary, Marks and Signs of the Triad, Yoni, Color of Gods, Fish and Good Friday, Tortoise, Earth Mother, Unity, Fourfold God, Meru, Religious Prostitution, Shaga, Communion Buns and Religious Cakes, Antiquity of the Cross, Crucifixion, Christna, Phallic and Sun Worship, The Phallus in California.

THE MESSAGE OF AQUARIA by Curtiss. The Mystic Life, The Sign Aquarius, Are These the Last Days?, Comets and Eclipses, Law of Growth, Birth of the New Age, Mastery and the Masters of Wisdom, Mother Earth and the Four Winds, The Spiral of Life and Life Waves, The Message of the Sphinx, Day of Judgement and Law of Sacrifice, The Spiritual Birth, The True Priesthood, Etc.

THE OCCULT ARTS by J.W. Frings. Alchemy, Astrology, Psychometry, Telepathy, Clairvoyance, Spiritualism, Hypnotism, Geomancy, Palmistry, Omens and Oracles.

THE OCCULT ARTS OF ANCIENT EGYPT by Bernard Bromage. Foreword, The Nature of the Ancient Egyptian Civilization, What the Ancient Egyptians Understood by Magic, The Destiny of the Soul According to the Egyptians, Egyptian Magic and Belief in Amulets and Talismans, The Egyptian Magicians, Black Magic in Ancient Egypt, The Astrological Implications of Egyptian Magic, Ancient Egypt and the Universal Dream Life, (Includes Various Illustrations).

OCCULTISTS & MYSTICS OF ALL AGES by Ralph Shirley. Apollonius of Tyana, Plotinus, Michael Scot, Paracelsus, Emanuel Swedenborg, Count Cagliostro, Anna Kingsford.

SEMA-KANDA: THRESHOLD MEMORIES by Coulson Turnbull. Ra-Om-Ar and Sema-Kanda, The Brotherhood, Sema-Kanda's Childhood, The Scroll, Posidona, Questioning, Ramantha's Lesson, The Great White Lodge, The Destruction of Atlantis, The Two Prisoners, The Congregation of the Inquisition, An Invitation, A Musical Evening, Two Letters, Confidences, The Horoscope, Etc.

VOICE OF ISIS by H.A. & F.A. Curtiss. Life's Duties, The Cycle of Fulfillment, Degrees and Orders, The Wisdom Religion, Concerning the Doctrine of Hell Fire, The Eleventh Commandment, Narcotics, Alcohol and Phychism, A Study of Karma, The Self, The Doctrine of Avatara, The Study of Reincarnation, Power, A Brief Outline of Evolution, The Laws, World Chains, Purity, The Origin of Man, The Symbol of the Serpent, Purification vs Deification, The Memory of Past Lives, The Cycle of Necessity, Etc!

WHAT IS OCCULTISM? by Papus. Occultism Defined, Occult Philosophical Point of View, Ethics of Occultism, Aesthetics of Occultism, Theodicy – Sociology, Practice of Occultism, The Traditions of Magic, Occultism and Philosophy.

YOUR UNSEEN GUIDE by C.J. Halsted. The Manner in Which You are Guided, How I Am Guided Consciously, Omens, The Intermediate State, Heaven, Spiritualism, The "Spirit Man" Illusion Dispelled, Evidence of My Guide's Prescience, Evolution.

GRAPHOLOGY

HOW TO READ CHARACTER IN HANDWRITING by Mary H. Booth. Principles of Analysis and Deduction, Forming Impressions from the Handwriting, The Autograph Fad, Entertaining by Graphology, Graphology as a Profession, Index.

HEALING

DIVINE REMEDIES – A TEXTBOOK ON CHRISTIAN HEALING by Theodosia DeWitt Schobert. Fuller Understanding of Spiritual Healing, Healing of Blood Troubles and Skin Diseases, Freedom from Sense Appetite, Healing of Insanity, Healing of Insomnia, Healing of Poisoning of Any Kind, General Upbuilding and Healing of the Body Temple.

THE FINER FORCES OF NATURE IN DIAGNOSIS AND THERAPY by George Starr White, M.D. The Magnetic Meridian, Vital and Unseen Forces, Polarity, Cause of Un-Health, Colors, Magnetic Energy, Sympathetic-Vagal Reflex, Actions of Finer Forces of Nature, The Human Aura, Moon-Light and Sound Treatment with Light and Color, Etc.

HEAL THYSELF: AN EXPLANATION OF THE REAL CAUSE AND CURE OF DISEASE by Edward Bach, M.B., B.S., D.P.H. by focusing on the causes rather than the results of disease and thus allowing individuals to assist in their own healing, Dr. Bach shows the vital principles which will guide medicine in the near future and are indeed guiding some of the more advanced members of the profession today.

HEALTH AND SPIRITUAL HEALING by Richard Lynch. The Key to Health, Statements for the Realization of Health, Rhythm of Life and Health, The Revelation of the Body, Realizing the Perfect Body, The Tree of Life and Health, Establishing the Incorruptible Body, Health Personified, Bringing Forth the True Body, How to Renew Your Consciousness, Individual Rebirth in Consciousness, Individual Resurrection, Ideas for Individual Ressurection.

THE KEY TO MAGNETIC HEALING by J.H. Strasser. The History of Magnetic Healing, The Theory of Magnetic Healing, Proof of Its Existence, What it is, Sources of it, Are Vital Magnetism and Electricity the Same, Have all Persons Magnetic Power?, Mental Science, The Principle of Life in Man, Mind and Magnetism, The Will Power, Mind over Matter, Passivity or Hypnotism, Why is Suggestion so Effective during Passivity?, Telepathy, Experiments, Testing Susceptibility, To Find Hidden Objects, Producing the Passive State, Suggestion, Manipulation, and Passes, General Treatment by Suggestion, Producing Anaesthesia, Hypnotizing at a Distance, Suggestion during Common Sleep, Suggestion during Waking State, Telepathy or Mind—Telegraphy, The Practice of Magnetic Healing, Can Magnetic Healing be Suppressed?, Unconscious Magnetic Healing, Treatment of the Different Diseases, Nervous Diseases, Blood Diseases, caused by Congestion and Irregular Circulation, Miscellaneous Diseases, Etc!

THE PHILOSOPHY OF MENTAL HEALING – A PRACTICAL EXPOSITION OF NATURAL RESTORATIVE POWER by Leander Edmund Whipple. Metaphysical Healing, Metaphysics Versus Hypnotism, The Potency of Metaphysics in Surgery, The Progress of the Age, Intelligence and Sensation, Mental Action, The Physical Reflection of Thought.

THE PRINCIPLES OF OCCULT HEALING Edited by Mary Weeks Burnett, M.D. Occult Healing and Occultism, Healing and the Healing Intelligence. The Indestructible Self, Latent Powers of Matter, The Auras and the Ethers, Polarization, Music, Healing by Prayer, Angel or Deva Helpers, Thought Forms and Color in Healing, Magnetism – Mesmerism, Healing Miracles of the Christ, Etc

THE TWELVE HEALERS AND OTHER REMEDIES by Edward Bach. Chapters include remedies for the following: For Fear, For Uncertainty, For Insufficient Interest in Present Circumstances, For Loneliness, For Those Over-Sensitive to Influences and Ideas, For Despondency or Despair, For Over-Care for Welfare of Others.

HERBS

THE COMPLETE HERBALIST or THE PEOPLE THEIR OWN PHYSICIANS by Dr. O. Phelps Brown. By the use of Nature's Remedies great curative properties found in the Herbal Kingdom are described. A New and Plain System of Hygienic Principles Together with Comprehensive Essays on Sexual Philosophy, Marriage, Divorce, Etc.

THE TRUTH ABOUT HERBS by Mrs. C.F. Loyd. The Unbroken Tradition of Herbal Medicine, The History of Herbalism, The Birth of the Society of Herbalists, Herbs Cure-The Reason Why, The Healing Properties of Certain Herbs, The Effect of Herbs on Allergic Diseases, Herbalists' Fight for Freedom, Etc.

HISTORICAL NOVEL

CHILD OF THE SUN: A HISTORICAL NOVEL by Frank Cheavens. Alvar Nuñez Cabeza de Vaca was the first European explorer to cross the North American continent. His early 16th century wandering took him across Texas, part of New Mexico, southeastern Arizona, and down the west coast of Mexico into South America. His altruistic work and healing ministrations among the Indians of the Southwest drew to him multitudes of Indians who revered him as the Child of the Sun. Here, his story is told through the eyes of a deformed, itinerant Pueblo trader who joined him, studied with him, and witnessed the Great Spirit working through him.

HOLLOW EARTH

ETIDORHPA or THE END OF EARTH by John Uri Lloyd. Journey toward the center of the Earth thru mighty mushroom forests and across huge underground oceans with an entire series of fantastic experiences. A true occult classic! "Etidorhpa, the End of Earth, is in all respects the worthiest presentation of occult teachings under the attractive guise of fiction that has yet been written" – New York World.

BEING AND BECOMING - THE PRINCIPLES AND PRACTICES OF THE SCIENCE OF SPIRIT by Fenwicke L. Holmes. The Impersonal Mind, Becoming, Allowing Mind to Act, Unconscious Activity,The Great Law of Mind, The Law of Correspondence, Picturing our Good, Ideataion, Concentration vs. Ideation, Denials, Affirmation, Consciousness, A Healing Realization, The Personal Spirit, The Purpose of Spirit, The Motive - Love, Love Defined, Making our Unity, Love - The Healing Power, Feelings and Emotions, Why Many Fail, Mysticism, Our Power of Choice, Being, Intuition, Spirit as Formative, A Way to Escape, Identity with Spirit, Demonstrating Prosperity, The Law of Spirit, Mental Equivalents, Selling a House, Spirit as All, "I am He".

CHARACTER BUILDING THOUGHT POWER by Ralph Waldo Trine. "Have we within our power to determine at all times what types of habits shall take form in our lives? In other words, is habit-forming, character-building, a matter of mere chance, or do we have it within our control?"

CREATIVE MIND by Ernest S. Holmes. Chapters include: In the Beginning, Why and What is a Man?, The Law of Our Lives, Bondage and Freedom, The Word, The Power We Have Within Us, The Reason for the Universe, Mind in Action, Action and Reaction, Arriving at High Consciousness, The Perfect Universe, About Struggle Karma, Etc.

CRISIS IN CONSCIOUSNESS: The Source of All Conflict by Robert Powell. The Importance of Right Beginning, Zen and Liberation, The Worldly Mind and the Religious Mind, Repetition of the Pattern, Experience, Habit and Freedom, Can Illumination be Transmitted? The Equation of Unhappiness, Must We Have Religious Societies? Approach to the Immeasurable, Window on Non-Duality, Memory Without a Cause, Self or Non-Self? Common Sayings Revealing Uncommon Insights, On Contradiction, The Outer and the Inner, Etc.

THE FAITH THAT HEALS (HOW TO DEVELOP) by Fenwicke L. Holmes The New Consciousness, Cosmic Consciousness, The Law of Consciousness Outlines, Practical Use of Visions – Visualizing Prosperity and Health, the Cure of Organic Disease and "Incurables," New Healing and Prosperity Consciousness, Your Healing Word, Faith in Yourself, Developing Self-Confidence, etc.

THE FREE MIND: THE INWARD PATH TO LIBERATION by Robert Powell. Liberation and Duality, Crisis in Consciousness, Our Predicament, On Mindfulness, Living in the Essential, A Noncomparative Look at Zen and Krishnamurti, The Problem of Ambition, Only the Empty Mind is Capable of True Thoughtfulness, What Education Should Be All About, and What it Actually Is, If Awareness is Choiceless, Then Who is it That is Aware?, Free Among the Unfree, The Vicious, Vicious Circle of Self-Defense and War, Reflections on Causality: The Ultimate Failure of Metaphysics, Etc.

HEALTH AND WEALTH FROM WITHIN by William E. Towne. Health From Within, Awakening of the Soul, Will, Love and Work, The Voice of Life, Non-Attachment, The Woman – The Man, The Supreme Truth, Power of Imagination and Faith, Practical Self-Healing, The Way to Gain Results, Lengthen and Brighten Life, Etc.

ON THE OPEN ROAD - BEING SOME THOUGHTS AND A LITTLE CREED OF WHOLESOME LIVING by Ralph Waldo Trine. To realize always clearly, that thoughts are forces, that like creates like and like attracts like, and that to determine one's thinking therefore is to determine his life.

POSITIVE THOUGHTS ATTRACT SUCCESS by Mary A. Dodson and Ella E. Dodson. "Unless Your Heart Sings The Word, It Would Be Better Left Unuttered." "Unless We Can Do The Work Better, We Have No Right To Find Fault When Another Does It." "I Am a Holy Temple, and Send Out Love and Good To All The World." "What You Accomplish is Often Determined by What You Attempt." "I Will to go on From Strength to Strength, From Character to Character, Until I Have Developed a Powerful Personality."

SO SPEAKS HIGHER POWER: A HANDBOOK FOR EMOTIONAL AND SPIRITUAL RECOVERY by Dr. Isaac Shamaya. Addiction, Stress and Recovery, Feeling, Blame, Anger, Fear and Pain, Relationships, Understanding, Love, and Higher Power.

THE SUCCESS PROCESS by Brown Landone. Five Factors Which Guarantee Success. The Process of Vivid Thinking, Tones Used in Persuading, Use of Action, Overcoming Hindrances, Developing Capacities, Securing Justice, Augmenting Your Success by Leadership, Etc.

JAMES ALLEN TITLES

ABOVE LIFE'S TURMOIL by James Allen. True Happiness, The Immortal Man, The Overcoming of Self, The Uses of Temptation, The Man of Integrity, Discrimination, Belief, The Basis of Action, The Belief that Saves, Thought and Action, Your Mental Attitude, Sowing and Reaping, The Reign of Law, The Supreme Justice, The Use of Reason, Self-Discipline, Resolution, The Glorious Conquest, Contentment in Activity, The Temple of Brotherhood, Pleasant Pastures of Peace.

ALL THESE THINGS ADDED by James Allen. Entering the Kingdom, The Soul's Great Need, The Competitive Laws and the Law of Love, The Finding of a Principle, At Rest in the Kingdom, The Heavenly Life, The Divine Center, The Eternal Now, "The Original Simplicity", The Unfailing Wisdom, The Might of Meekness, The Righteous Man, Perfect Love, Greatness and Goodness, and Heaven in the Heart.

AS A MAN THINKETH by James Allen. Thought and Character, Effect of Thought on Circumstances, Effect of Thought on Health and the Body, Thought and Purpose, The Thought-Factor in Achievement, Visions and Ideals, Serenity.

BYWAYS OF BLESSEDNESS by James Allen. Right Beginnings, Small Tasks and Duties, Transcending Difficulties and Perplexities, Burden-Dropping, Hidden Sacrifices, Sympathy, Forgiveness, Seeing No Evil, Abiding Joy, Silentness, Solitude, Standing Alone, Understanding the Simple Laws of Life, Happy Endings.

EIGHT PILLARS OF PROSPERITY by James Allen. Discussion on Energy, Economy, Integrity, Systems, Sympathy, Sincerity, Impartiality, Self-reliance, and the Temple of Prosperity

ENTERING THE KINGDOM by James Allen. The Soul's Great Need, The Competitive Laws and the Laws of Love, The Finding of a Principle, At Rest in the Kingdom, And All Things Added.

FROM PASSION TO PEACE by James Allen. Passion, Aspiration, Temptation, Transmutation, Transcendence, Beatitude, Peace.

FROM POVERTY TO POWER by James Allen. Two books in one: The Path to Prosperity Including World a Reflex of Mental States, The Way Out of Undesirable Conditions, Silent Power of Thought, Controlling and Directing One's Forces, The Secret of Health, Success, and Power, Etc. and The Way of Peace including Power of Meditation, The Two Masters, Self and Truth, The Acquirement of Spiritual Power, Realization of Selfless Love, Entering into the Infinite, Perfect Peace, Etc.

THE HEAVENLY LIFE by James Allen. The Divine Center, The Eternal Now, The "Original Simplicity", The Unfailing Wisdom, The Might of Meekness, The Righteous Man, Perfect Love, Perfect Freedom, Greatness and Goodness, Heaven in the Heart.

THE LIFE TRIUMPHANT by James Allen. Faith and Courage, Manliness and Sincerity, Energy and Power, Self-Control and Happiness, Simplicity and Freedom, Right-Thinking and Repose, Calmness and Resource, Insight and Nobility, Man and the Master, and Knowledge and Victory.

LIGHT ON LIFE'S DIFFICULTIES by James Allen. The Light that Leads to Perfect Peace, Light on Facts and Hypotheses, The Law of Cause and Effect in Human Life, Values - Spiritual and Material, The Sense of Proportion, Adherence to Principle, The Sacrifice of the Self, The Management of the Mind, Self-Control: The Door of Heaven, Acts and their Consequences, The Way of Wisdom, Disposition, Individual Liberty, The Blessing and Dignity of Work, Good Manner and Refinement, Diversity of Creeds, Law and Miracle, War and Peace, The Brotherhood of Man, Life's Sorrows, Life's Change, The Truth of Transitoriness, The Light that Never Goes Out.

MAN: KING OF MIND, BODY AND CIRCUMSTANCE by James Allen. The Inner World of Thoughts, The Outer World of Things, Habit: Its Slavery and Its Freedom, Bodily Conditions, Poverty, Man's Spiritual Dominion, Conquest: Not Resignation.

THE MASTERY OF DESTINY by James Allen. Deeds, Character, and Destiny, The Science of Self-Control, Cause and Effect in Human Conduct, Training of the Will, Thoroughness, Mind-Building and Life-Building, Cultivation of Concentration, Practice of Meditation, The Power of Purpose, The Joy of Accomplishment.

MEDITATIONS, A YEAR BOOK by James Allen. "James Allen may truly be called the Prophet of Meditation. In an age of strife, hurry, religious controversy, heated arguments, ritual and ceremony, he came with his message of Meditation, calling men away from the din and strife of tongues into the peaceful paths of stillness within their own souls, where 'the Light that lighteth every man that cometh into the world' ever burns steadily and surely for all who will turn their weary eyes from the strife without to the quiet within." Contains two quotes and a brief commentary for each day of the year.

MORNING AND EVENING THOUGHTS by James Allen. Contains a separate and brief paragraph for each morning and evening of the month.

OUT FROM THE HEART by James Allen. The Heart and the Life, The Nature of Power of Mind, Formation of Habit, Doing and Knowing, First Steps in the Higher Life, Mental Conditions and Their Effects, Exhortation.

THROUGH THE GATE OF GOOD by James Allen. The Gate and the Way, The Law and the Prophets, The Yoke and the Burden, The Word and the Doer, The Vine and the Branches, Salvation this Day.

THE WAY OF PEACE by James Allen. The Power of Meditation, The Two Masters: Self and Truth, The Acquirement of Spiritual Power, The Realization of Selfless Love, Entering into the Infinite, Saints, Sages, and Saviors, The Law of Service, The Realization of Perfect Peace.

PERSONALITY: ITS CULTIVATION AND POWER AND HOW TO ATTAIN by Lily L. Allen. Personality, Right Belief, Self-Knowledge, Intuition, Decision and Promptness, Self-Trust, Thoroughness, Manners, Physical Culture, Mental, Moral, and Spiritual Culture, Introspection, Emancipation, Self-Development, Self-Control and Mental Poise, Liberty, Transformation, Balance, Meditation and Concentration.

KUNDALINI

AND THE SUN IS UP: KUNDALINI RISES IN THE WEST by W. Thomas Wolfe. Chapters include: The Hindu's View, The Esoteric Christian's View, The Professional Specialist's View, The Kundalini Subject's View, Physiological Effects, Spiritual Weightlessness, Emotional and Attitudinal Changes, Changed Dream Content, Event Control, The Reason for Summoning Up the Kundalini, Christ and the Kundalini, A Modern Parallel to the Second Coming, Etc.

LIGHT

PHILOSOPHY OF LIGHT – AN INTRODUCTORY TREATISE by Floyd Irving Lorbeer. The Ocean of Light, Sight and Light, Light and Perception, Some Cosmic Considerations, Light and Health, Electrical Hypothesis, Temperament, Beauty, and Love and Light, The Problem of Space and Time, Unity and Diversity, Deity, Soul, and Immortality, Light and the New Era, Etc.

PRINCIPLES OF LIGHT AND COLOR by Edwin D. Babbitt. (Illustrated, Complete 578p. version.) The Harmonic Laws of the Universe, The Etherio-Atomic Philosophy of Force, Chromo Chemistry, Chromo Therapeutics, and the General Philosophy of Finer Forces, Together with Numerous Discoveries and Practical Applications, Etc!

LONGEVITY

FOREVER YOUNG: HOW TO ATTAIN LONGEVITY by Gladys Iris Clark. Chapter include: Ageless Symbology, Followers of Fallen Luminaries, Rejuvenation Practices, Youth in Age-Old Wisdom, Angelic Travel Guides, Longevity Begins with God Awareness, Coping with Realities, Non-Aging Techniques in Action, Musing on Transition, Cancel Out Negatives, Grecian Nostalgia, Sedona's Seven Vortices, Crystals, Etc.

MEDITATION

CONCENTRATION AND MEDITATION by Christmas Humphreys. The Importance of Right Motive, Power of Thought, Dangers and Safeguards, Particular Exercises, Time, Place, Posture, Relaxation, Breathing, Thoughts, Counting the Breaths, Visualization and Color, Stillness, Motive, Self Analogy, Higher Meditation, The Voice of Mysticism, Jhanas, Zen, Satori, Koan, Ceremonial Magic, Taoism, Occultism, Mysticism, Theosophy, Yoga, The Noble Eightfold Path, Etc.

MYTHOLOGY

A DICTIONARY OF NON-CLASSICAL MYTHOLOGY by Marian Edwardes & Lewis Spence. An exceptional work! "Not one mythology, but several, will be found concentrated within the pages of this volume . . ." Covers everything from Aah (Ah): An Egyptian moon-god, thru Brigit: A goddess of the Irish Celts, Excalibur: King Arthur's Sword, Hou Chi: A Chinese divine personage, . . . Huitzilopochtli of the Aztecs . . . Mama Cocha of Peru . . . Uttu: The Sumerian . . . Valkyrie (Old German): Female warriors . . . Byelun: A white Russian deity, . . . Meke Meke: The god-creator of Easter Island, Mwari: The Great Spirit of the Mtawara tribe of Rhodesia, Triglav (Three heads): Baltic Slav deity. . . and hundreds more!

NEW THOUGHT

THE GIFT OF THE SPIRIT A Selection From the Essays of Prentice Mulford With Preface and Introduction by Arthur Edward Waite. The Infinite Mind in Nature, The God in Yourself, The Doctor Within & Mental Medicine, Faith or Being Led by the Spirit, The Material Mind vs. The Spiritual Mind, What are Spirtual Gifts?, Regeneration or Being Born Again, Re-Embodiment Universal in Nature, You Travel When You Sleep, Prayer In All Ages, Etc!

THE HEART OF THE NEW THOUGHT by Ella Wheeler Wilcox. Let the Past Go, The Sowing of the Seed, Thought Force, Opulence and Eternity, Morning Influences, The Philosophy of Happiness, Common Sense, Heredity and Invincibility, The Object of Life, Wisdom and Self Conquest, Concentration and Destiny, The Breath, Generosity and Balance, Etc!

THE HIDDEN POWER AND OTHER PAPERS UPON MENTAL SCIENCE by Thomas Troward. The Hidden Power, The Perversion of Truth, The "I Am", Affirmative Power, The Principle of Guidance, Desire as the Motive Power, Touching Lightly, The Spirit of Opulence, Beauty, Seperation and Unity, Entering into the Spirit of It, The Bible and New Thought, What is Higher Thought?, Etc!

THE LAW OF THE NEW THOUGHT by Willam Walker Atkinson. What is the New Thought?, Thoughts are Things, The Law of Attraction, Mind Building, The Dweller of the Threshold, Mind and Body, The Mind and its Planes, The Subconsious Plane, The Super-Conscious Faculties, The Soul's Question, The Absolute, The Oneness of All, The Immortality of the Soul, The Unfoldment, The Growth of Consciouness, The Soul's Awakening.

THOUGHT FORCES by Prentice Mulford. Chapters include: Co-operation of Thought, Some Practical Mental Recipes, The Drawing Power of Mind, Buried Talents, The Necessity of Riches, The Uses of Sickness, The Doctor Within, Mental Medicine, The Use and Necessity of Recreation, The Art of Forgetting, Cultivate Repose, Love Thyself.

THOUGHTS ARE THINGS by Prentice Mulford. The Material Mind vs. The Spiritual Mind, Who Are Our Relations?, Thought Currents, One Way to Cultivate Courage, Look Forward, God in the Trees, Some Laws of Health and Beauty, Museum and Menagerie Horrors, The God in Yourself, Healing and Renewing Force of Spring, Immorality in the Flesh, Attraction of Aspiration, The Accession of New Thought.

NUMEROLOGY

NAMES, DATES, AND NUMBERS – A SYSTEM OF NUMEROLOGY by Roy Page Walton. The Law of Numbers, The Character and influence of the Numbers, Application and Use of Numbers, Strong and Weak Names. The Number that Governs the Life, How Each Single Name Effects the Life, The Importance of Varying the Signature, How the Name Discloses the Future, Choosing a Suitable Name for a Child, Names Suitable for Marriage, How to Find Lucky Days and Months, Points to Bear in Mind.

NUMBERS: THEIR OCCULT POWER AND MYSTIC VIRTUE by W. Wynn Wescott. Pythagoras, His Tenets and His Followers, Pythagorean Views of Numbers, Kabalistic View on Numbers, Properties of the Numbers according to the Bible, the Talmuds, the Pythagoreans, the Romans, Chaldeans, Egyptians, Hindoos, Medieval Magicians, Hermetic Students, and the Rosicurcians.

NUMBER VIBRATION IN QUESTIONS AND ANSWERS by Mrs. L. Dow Balliett. Selections include: When Was Your First Birth?, The First Step in Reading a Name, Can the Name be Changed?, What Does the Birth Path Show?, The Numerical and Number Chart, Is an Esoteric Value to be Found in Gems?, Why Do We Not Add Either 22 or 11?, The Day of Reincarnation, Is Anybody Out of Place?, Are We Gods?, Of What Use is Prayer?, What Is the Soul?, Should Rooms be Furnished in our Own Colors?, What Months Are Best for Creation?, What Is Astral Music?, Where Should We Live?, Etc. Etc. Etc!

NUMERAL PHILOSOPHY by Albert Christy. A Study of Numeral Influences upon the Physical, Mental, and Spiritual Nature of Mankind.

VIBRATION: A SYSTEM OF NUMBERS AS TAUGHT BY PYTHARGORAS by Mrs. L. Dow Balliett. Chapters include: The Principles of Vibration, Numbers in Detail, What Your Name Means (broadly speaking), Business, Choosing A Husband or Wife, Pythagoras' Laws, Your Colors, Body Parts, Gems, Minerals, Flowers, Birds, Odors, Music, Guardian Angel, Symbols, Etc.

ORIENTAL (Also see "YOGA")

THE BUDDHA'S GOLDEN PATH by Dwight Goddard. Prince Siddhartha Gautama, Right Ideas, Speech, Behaviour, Right Vocation, Words, Conduct, Mindfulness, Concentration, Resolution, Environment, Intuition, Vows, Radiation, Spiritual Behaviour, Spirit, Etc.

BUSHIDO: WAY OF THE SAMURAI Translated from the classic Hagakure by Minoru Tanaka. This unique translation of a most important Japanese classic offers an explanation of the central and upright character of the Japanese people, and their indomitable inner strength. "The Way of the Samurai" is essential for businessmen, lawyers, students, or anyone who would understand the Japanese psyche.

DAO DE JING (LAO-ZI): THE OLD SAGE'S CLASSIC OF THE WAY OF VIRTUE translated by Patrick Michael Byrne. A new translation, faithful to both the letter and the poetic spirit of the original, of the ancient Chinese book of wisdom (traditionally known as the *Tao Te Ching* of Lao Tse or Lao Tsu: this version employs the new, more accurate *pinyin* transliteration). With introduction, notes and commentary.

FUSANG or THE DISCOVERY OF AMERICA BY CHINESE BUDDHIST PRIESTS IN THE FIFTH CENTURY by Charles G. Leland. Chinese Knowledge of Lands and Nations, The Road to America, The Kingdom of Fusang or Mexico, Of Writing and Civil Regulations in Fusang, Laws and Customs of the Aztecs, The Future of Eastern Asia, Travels of Other Buddhist Priests, Affinities of American and Asiatic Languages, Images of Buddha, Etc.

THE HISTORY OF BUDDHIST THOUGHT by Edward J. Thomas. The Ascetic Ideal, Early Doctrine: Yoga, Brahminism and the Upanishads, Karma, Release and Nirvana, Buddha, Popular Bodhisattva Doctrine, Buddhism and Modern Thought, Etc.

THE IMITATION OF BUDDHA - QUOTATIONS FROM BUDDHIST LITERATURE FOR EACH DAY OF THE YEAR Compiled by Ernest M. Bowden with preface by Sir Edwin Arnold. These 366 wonderful quotes are taken from a broad base of Buddhist Literature including many now hard-to-find texts.

SACRED BOOKS OF THE EAST by Epiphanius Wilson. Vedic Hymns, The Zend-Avesta, The Dhammapada, The Upanishads, Selections from the Koran, Life of Buddha, Etc.

THE WISDOM OF THE HINDUS by Brian Brown. Brahmanic Wisdom, Maha-Bharata, The Ramayana, Wisdom of the Upanishads, Vivekananda and Ramakrishna on Yoga Philosophy, Wisdom of Tuka-Ram, Paramananda, Vivekananda, Abbedananda, Etc.

PALMISTRY

INDIAN PALMISTRY by Mrs. J.B. Dale. A Summary of Judgement, Signification of Animals, Flowers, and Promiscuous Marks Found on the Hand, The Lines, The Mounts, The Line of Life, The Events, The Line of the Head and Brain, The Line of Fortune, Saturn, Venus and Mars, The Rule to Tell The Planets, The Mount of Jupiter, Apollo the Sun, The Moon, The Mount of Saturn , The Planet Mercury, Mensa: The Part of Fortune, The Fingers and Thumb, The Head and Signs of the Feet, The Arms, Etc.

PHILOSOPHY

GOETHE – WITH SPECIAL CONSIDERATION OF HIS PHILOSOPHY by Paul Carus. The Life of Goethe, His Relation to Women, Goethe's Personality, The Religion of Goethe, Goethe's Philosophy, Literature and Criticism, The Significance of "Faust", Miscellaneous Epigrams and Poems. (Heavily Illustrated).

PROPHECY (Also See Earth Changes)

THE STORY OF PROPHECY by Henry James Forman. What is Prophecy?, Oracles, The Great Pyramid Speaks, The End of the Age: Biblical Prophecy, Medieval Prophecy, Astrologers and Saints, Prophecies Concerning the Popes, Nostradamus, America In Prophecy, The Prophetic Future.

PYRAMIDOLOGY

THE GREAT PYRAMID. Two Essays plus illustrations, one from The Reminder and the other from J.F. Rowney Press. Selections include: The Pyramid's Location and Constructional Features, Some of the Pyramid's Scientific Features, other Features of the Great Pyramid, Complete History of Mankind Represented in the Pyramid, The Shortening of Time, The Symbolism of the Passages and Chambers, Etc.

THE GREAT PYRAMID - Its Construction, Symbolism, and Chronology by Basil Stewart. Construction and Astrological Features, Chart of World History, Missing Apexstone, Who Built It? Plus Various Diagrams.

REINCARNATION

LIFE AFTER LIFE: THE THEORY OF REINCARNATION by Eustace Miles. Have We Lived Before? Questions Often Asked, Does Not Oppose Christianity, Great Men Who Have Believed, etc.

THE NEW REVELATION by Sir Arthur Conan Doyle. The Search, The Revelation, The Coming Life, Problems and Limitations, The Next Phase of Life, Automatic Writing, The Cheriton Dugout.

REINCARNATION by George B. Brownell. He Knew Who He Was, Memories of Past Lives, A Remarkable Proof, Lived Many Lives, An Arabian Incarnation, Dreamed of Past Life, Great Minds and Reincarnation, The Bible and Reincarnation, Karma, Atlantis Reborn, Thought is Destiny, The Celestial Body, The Hereafter, Etc.

REINCARNATION by F. Homer Curtiss, M.D. The Doctrine, Why and How, In the New Testament, Objections Answered, Scientific Evidence and Physical Proof.

REINCARNATION by Katherine Tingley. What Reincarnation Is, Arguments for Reincarnation, Supposed Objections to Reincarnation, Reincarnation and Heredity, Reincarnation in Antiquity, Reincarnation the Master-Key to Modern Problems, Reincarnation In Modern Literature.

THE RING OF RETURN by Eva Martin. Pre-Christian Era, Early Christian and Other Writings of the First Five Centuries A.D., Miscellaneous Sources Before A.D. 1700, A.D. 1700-1900, The Twentieth Century. In this book, Miss Eva Martin has brought together a most complete and scholarly collection of references to past, present, and future life.

RELIGIONS

THE BIBLE IN INDIA - Hindoo Origin of Hebrew and Christian Revelation Translated from "La Bible Dans L'Inde" by Louis Jacolliot. India's Relation to Antiquity, Manou, Manes, Minos, Moses, What the Lessons of History are Worth, Brahminical Perversions of Primitive Vedism, Virgins of the Pagodas and Rome, Moses or Moise and Hebrew Society, Zeus - Jezeus - Isis - Jesus, Moses Founds Hebrew Society on the Model of Egypt and India, The Hindoo Genesis, Zeus and Brahma, Devas and Angels, The Hindoo Trinity, Adima (In Sanscrit, The First Man), Ceylon as the Garden of Paradise, The Woman of the Vedas and The Woman of the Bible, The Deluge According to the Maha-Barata, Prophecies Announcing the Coming of Christna, Birth of the Virgin Devanaguy, Massacre of all Male Children Born on the Same Night as Christna, Christna Begins to Preach the New Law, His Disciples, Parable of the Fisherman, Christna's Philosophic Teaching, Transfiguration of Christna, His Disiples Give Him The Name of Jezeus (Pure Essence), Christna and the Two Holy Women, Death of Christna, Hindoo Origin of the Christian Idea, Devanaguy and Mary, Christna and Christ, Massacre of the Innocents in India and Judea, Hindoo and Christian Transfiguration, Apocrypha of St. John, Whence the Monks and Hermits of Primitive Christianity, A Text of Manou, Etc!

NATURAL LAW IN THE SPIRITUAL WORLD by Henry Drummond. Biogenesis, Degeneration, Growth, Death, Mortification, Eternal Life, Environment, Conformity to Type, Semi-Parasitism, Parasitism, Classification.

PRINCIPAL SYMBOLS OF WORLD RELIGIONS by Swami Harshananda. Chapters include discussions of the symbols of these religions: Hinduism, Buddhism, Jainism, Sikhism, Shintoism, Islam, Christianity, Judaism, Zoroastrianism, Taoism.

THE RELIGION OF THE SIKH GURUS by Teja Singh, M.A., Teja Singh, formerly a professor of history at Khalsa College in Amritsar, outlines the foundation of history, tradition, ritual and principles which has kept disciples of the the Sikh religion strong and united into the present day.

SELF-HELP / RECOVERY (See under "Inspiration, etc.")

SOUL

THE HUMAN SOUL IN SLEEPING, DREAMING AND WAKING by F.W. Zeylmans van Emmichoven, M.D. Featured subjects include: What is the Soul?, How, by observing the phenomena of life, we can find the reality of the soul and its connections with the human organism. Man as a threefold being. Dreams. Psycho-Analysis. The awakening of the soul. Fears. Meditation, Concentration and Self Development. The counterforces that work against man's spiritual striving. Spiritual Science as a psychology of the living, developing soul, Etc.

THE INNER MAN by Hanna Hurnard. A Parable, The Inner Man, Communication with the Heavenly World, The Soul of the Inner Man, The Garments of the Soul, Soul Disease and Soul Healing, The Soul's Psychic Powers, The Mystic Way.

TAROT

THE ILLUSTRATED KEY TO THE TAROT – THE VEIL OF DIVINATION by Arthur Edward Waite. The Veil and Its Symbols, The Tarot in History, The Doctrine Behind the Veil, The Outer Method of the Oracles, The Four Suits of Tarot Cards, The Art of Tarot Divination, An Ancient Celtic Method of Divination.

THE KEY OF DESTINY by H.A. and F.H. Curtiss. The Initiate, Twelve-fold Division of the Zodiac, Reincarnation and Transmutation, The Solar System, The Letters of the Tarot, The Numbers 11 thru 22, Twelve Tribes and Twelve Disciples, The Great Work, The Labors of Hercules, Necromancy, Great Deep, Temperance, Man the Creator vs. the Devil, Celestial Hierarchies, The New Jerusalem, Etc.

THE KEY TO THE UNIVERSE by H.A. and F.H. Curtiss. Origin of the Numerical Systems, Symbols of the "O" as the Egg and the Cat, The "O" as the Aura and the Ring Pass Not, Symbol of the O, Letters of the Tarot, The Numbers 1 thru 10, The 7 Principles of Man, The 7 Pleiades and the 7 Rishis, Joy of Completion.

WESTERN MYSTICISM

ANCIENT MYSTERY AND MODERN REVELATION by W.J. Colville. Rivers of Life or Faiths of Man in All Lands, Ancient and Modern Ideas of Revelation - Its Sources and Agencies, Creation Legends - How Ancient is Humanity On this Planet? Egypt and Its Wonders: Literally and Mystically Considered, The Philosophy of Ancient Greece, The School of Pythagoras, The Delphic Mysteries, Apollonius of Tyana, Five Varieties of Yoga, Union of Eastern and Western Philosophy, Ezekiel's Wheel - What it Signifies, The Book of Exodus - Its Practical and Esoteric Teachings, The Message of Buddhism - Purity and Philanthropy, Magic in Europe in the Middle Ages, Ancient Magic and Modern Therapeutics, Bible Symbolism, The Law of Seven and the Law of Unity, The Esoteric Teachings of the Gnostics.

BROTHERHOOD OF MT. SHASTA by Eugene E. Thomas. From Clouds to Sunshine, Finding the Brotherhood, The Lake of Gold, The Initiation, Memories of the Past, In Advance of the Future, Prodigy, Trial, and Visitor, The Annihilation and the King, The Lost Lemuria.

CLOTHED WITH THE SUN - BEING THE BOOK OF THE ILLUMINATIONS OF ANNA (BONUS) KINGSFORD Edited by Edward Maitland and Samuel Hopgood Hart. Concerning the three Veils between Man and God, The Powers of the Air, The Devil and Devils, The Gods, Psyche; or the Human Soul, Dying, The Mysteries of God, The Divine Image; or the Vision of Adonai, Etc.

INNER RADIANCE by H.A. & F.A. Curtiss. The Inner Radiance, Spiritual Co-operation, Man and the Zodiac, The Soul-Language, Transmigration, Cosmic Cause of World Conditions, Planetary and Karmic Factors, The Mystic Rose, The Lords of Karma, The Great Works, The Mystery of the Elements, The Third Eye, The Round Table, The Ancient Continents, Nature's Symbology.

KALEVALA: THE LAND OF THE HEROES Translated by W. F. Kirby. The National Epic of Finland. "...the Kalevala itself could one day becomes as important for all of humanity as Homer was for the Greeks."

THE FOUR GREAT INITIATIONS, by Ellen Conroy M.A. Foreward by Leon Dabo, Initiation by Water, The Mystical Understanding of Baptism, Temptation, The Power of the Spirit, Initiation by Air, The Mystical Understanding of the Plucking of Corn on the Sabbath Day, The Sermon on the Mount, Initiation by Fire, The Transfiguration, Initiation by Earth, The Crucifiction and Ascension.

MYRIAM AND THE MYSTIC BROTHERHOOD by Maude Lesseuer Howard. A novel in the western mystic tradition.

THE WAY OF ATTAINMENT by Sydney T. Klein. The Invisible is the Real, The Power of Prayer, Spiritual Regeneration, Dogma of the Virgin Birth, Finding the Kingdom of Heaven "Within", Realizing Oneness with God, Nature of the Ascent, Reaching the Summit.

THE WAY OF MYSTICISM by Joseph James. God Turns Towards Man, The Unexpected, The Still Small Voice, His Exceeding Brightness, Man Turns Towards God, The Obstructive "Me", Where East and West Unite, Beside the Still Waters, Love's Meeting Place, Work – A Prayer, Every Pilgrim's Progress, Love's Fulfillment.

TABLOID MAGAZINE The Astral Projection. Metaphysical Tabloid Magazine from the early 1970's. Last three issues available.

YOGA (also see ORIENTAL)

YOGA PHILOSOPHY AND PRACTICE by Hari Prasad Shastri. The History and Literature of Yoga, The Epics and Bhagavad Gita, Patanjali, Shankaracharya, The Philosophy of Yoga, The Vedanta, Reason and Intuition, The Teacher (Guru), Advita (Non-Dualism), God and the World, God (Brahman) and the Individual (Jiva), The Nature of the Self, The Personal God (Ishvara), Three Views of Maya, The Three Gunas, Ethics, Action (Karma), Death and Reincarnation, Liberation, The Practice of Yoga, Subjects for Meditation, Peace of Mind, The True Self, Dream and Sleep, Vital Currents of the Body, OM, Practice in Daily Life, Austerity, Posture, Pranayama (Control of the Vital Currents), Concentration, Contemplation (Dhyana), Samadhi, Liberation in Life, Practical Program, Obstructions, Common Sense in Training, The Process in Brief, Three Yogis, Rama Tirtha, Shri Dada, Kobo Daishi, Illustrative Passages from the Literature of Yoga, Prayers from the Vedas, The Upanishads, The Bhagavad Gita, Yoga Vasishtha, The Ashtavakra Gita, Poem by Swami Rama Tirtha, Glossary, Etc!

GENERAL NON-METAPHYSICAL

BEST ENGRAVINGS by Skip Whitson. One hundred twenty three beautiful steel cut and wood cut engravings from the nineteenth century.

BUSTED IN MEXICO by Ann Palmer and Jessica Herman. One young woman's story of the devastating effects of the loss of liberty. A True Story, Introduction by Governor Jerry Apodaca.

THE LAND OF ENCHANTMENT FROM PIKE'S PEAK TO THE PACIFIC by Lilian Whiting. Chapters include: With Western Stars and Sunsets, Denver the Beautiful, The Picturesque Region of Pike's Peak, Summer Wanderings in Colorado, The Colorado Pioneers, The Surprises of New Mexico, The Story of Santa Fe, Magic and Mystery of Arizona, The Petrified Forest and the Meteorite Mountain, Los Angeles, The Spell-Binder, Grand Canyon, the Carnival of the Gods.

SUN HISTORICAL SERIES 33 titles ranging from Maine 100 years ago to Hawaii 100 years ago.

MAYDAYS AND MERMAIDS by William A. Davis. A contemporary tale of the sea. Vivid fast moving satirical yarn, spun on the paradoxical spool of tragicomedy. "Once you start this book there is a high probability that you will not put it down." - Clark Chambers, Critic.

For a PRICE LIST of all currently available Sun Books titles write: Book List, Sun Publishing Co., P.O. Box 5588, Santa Fe, NM 87502-5588